O A O L
OXFORD AMERICAN ONCOLOGY LIBRARY

Renal Cell Carcinoma

O A O L
OXFORD AMERICAN ONCOLOGY LIBRARY

Renal Cell Carcinoma

Edited by

Nizar M. Tannir, MD, FACP

Professor and Deputy Chair
Department of Genitourinary Medical Oncology
Division of Cancer Medicine
The University of Texas MD Anderson Cancer Center
Houston, Texas

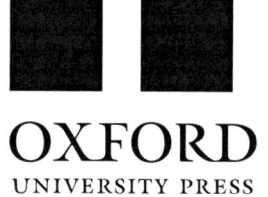

OXFORD
UNIVERSITY PRESS

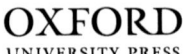

OXFORD
UNIVERSITY PRESS

Oxford University Press is a department of the University of Oxford.
It furthers the University's objective of excellence in research, scholarship,
and education by publishing worldwide.

Oxford   New York
Auckland   Cape Town   Dar es Salaam   Hong Kong   Karachi
Kuala Lumpur   Madrid   Melbourne   Mexico City   Nairobi
New Delhi   Shanghai   Taipei   Toronto

With offices in
Argentina   Austria   Brazil   Chile   Czech Republic   France   Greece
Guatemala   Hungary   Italy   Japan   Poland   Portugal   Singapore
South Korea   Switzerland   Thailand   Turkey   Ukraine   Vietnam

Oxford is a registered trademark of Oxford University Press
in the UK and certain other countries.

Published in the United States of America by
Oxford University Press
198 Madison Avenue, New York, NY 10016

Library of Congress Cataloging-in-Publication Data

Renal cell carcinoma (Tannir)
Renal cell carcinoma / edited by Nizar M. Tannir.
p. ; cm.—(Oxford American oncology library)
Includes bibliographical references and index.
ISBN 978–0–19–998813–6 (alk. paper)
I. Tannir, Nizar M., editor.   II. Title.   III. Series: Oxford American oncology library.
[DNLM: 1. Carcinoma, Renal Cell.   2. Kidney Neoplasms.   3. Molecular Targeted
Therapy—methods. WJ 358]
RC280.K5
616.99′461—dc23
2014010925

This book is dedicated to our patients who inspire us every day and remind us of the urgency of our research to make renal cell cancer history and to Zita Dubauskas Lim for her unwavering support and advocacy for our patients.

vi

Preface

The clinical care of the patient with renal cell carcinoma (RCC) has become increasingly complex. The incidence of RCC is increasing, in part, because of the wide use of modern imaging studies and, in part, because of the epidemic of obesity and dietary changes. Patients with RCC who have small renal masses have a spectrum of therapeutic options, ranging from active surveillance to high-energy ablation to nephron-sparing nephrectomy. For patients who present with locally advanced or metastatic disease, a multidisciplinary approach is essential for optimal management. Surgeons and medical oncologists are called upon to work as a team to incorporate systemic therapy and nephrectomy or metastasectomy. The optimal management of patients with RCC also requires the expertise of physicians from other disciplines including pathology, radiology, radiation oncology, pain management, and supportive care, as well as internal medicine and surgical subspecialties. Integrative oncology, which incorporates complementary and alternative medicine approaches, is emerging as a discipline to address the needs of patients with cancer who now use complementary medicines.

Insights into the biology of RCC, much gleaned from studies of inherited RCC syndromes, have led to the approval of seven molecularly targeted agents by the US Food and Drug Administration since December 2005, and more agents are on the horizon. The elucidation of von Hippel–Lindau gene dysregulation in clear-cell RCC and its impact on downstream targets, particularly the vascular endothelial growth factor (VEGF) pathway, have established anti-VEGF agents as bona fide therapies in metastatic clear-cell RCC. Agents that block the mammalian target of rapamycin pathway have also benefited patients with metastatic RCC. While more effective than interferon-alpha and less toxic than high-dose interleukin (IL)-2, targeted agents produce acute and chronic adverse events that may be challenging for long-term use. Although it has a formidable acute toxicity, high-dose IL-2 remains an option for a select few patients with metastatic clear-cell RCC and yields a 5% cure rate.

Despite the scientific progress made so far, which has led to improved progression-free survival and overall survival rates, the majority of patients with metastatic RCC will ultimately develop progressive disease and succumb to their cancer. Thus, research efforts are urgently needed to identify mechanisms of resistance to targeted agents and biomarkers of anti-tumor response and toxicity associated with these therapies. A concerted research effort is also needed to focus on discovery of relevant targets in RCC of variant histologies with suboptimal response to targeted agents.

Today, the science of oncology is witnessing a revolution in the way we think of cancer. Genomic medicine has ushered in a new era to tackle the cancer problem that cuts across traditional anatomic boundaries. Cancer immunotherapy is undergoing a renaissance with the development of immune checkpoint blockade therapies that unleash the full power of the immune system to attack cancer cells, regardless of their cell of origin or molecular type. The intersection of genomic medicine and immunotherapy will undoubtedly accelerate the pace of discovery toward the development of more effective treatments for "polygenic" cancers that have traditionally been resistant to chemotherapy and radiation.

The future of oncology has arrived. In this context, we present this book on RCC, a timely addition to the Oxford American Oncology Library. Our hope is that this concise book will bring to busy clinicians and trainees interested in RCC the knowledge and experience of leaders in the field who contributed to this book. Ultimately, our hope is for a future free of cancer.

Nizar M. Tannir, MD, FACP

Contents

Contributors

Michael B. Atkins, MD
Deputy Director and Chair
Department of Oncology
Georgetown-Lombardi
    Comprehensive Cancer Center
Division of Hematology/Oncology
Medstar Georgetown University
    Hospital
Washington, DC

Bradley Atkinson, PharmD, BCPS
Manager of Clinical Pharmacy
    Services
Department of Genitourinary
    Medical Oncology
The University of Texas MD
    Anderson Cancer Center
Houston, Texas

Diana Cauley, PharmD, BCOP
Clinical Pharmacy Specialist
Department of Genitourinary
    Medical Oncology
The University of Texas MD
    Anderson Cancer Center
Houston, Texas

Alejandro Chaoul, PhD
Assistant Professor
Director of Education, Integrative
    Medicine Program
General Oncology
The University of Texas MD
    Anderson Cancer Center
Houston, Texas

David D. Chism, MD, MS
Hematology/Oncology Fellow
University of North Carolina
Lineberger Cancer Center
Chapel Hill, North Carolina

Seungtaek Choi, MD
Assistant Professor
Department of Radiation Oncology
The University of Texas MD
    Anderson Cancer Center
Houston, Texas

Toni K. Choueiri, MD
Director, Kidney Cancer Center
Division of Medical Oncology
Dana Farber Cancer Institute
Brigham & Women's Hospital
Boston, Massachusetts

Wong-Ho Chow, PhD
Professor
Department of Epidemiology
The University of Texas MD
    Anderson Cancer Center
Houston, Texas

Lorenzo Cohen, PhD
Professor of Oncology
Director of Integrative Medicine
    Program
The University of Texas MD
    Anderson Cancer Center
Houston, Texas

Ruhee Dere, PhD
Assistant Professor
Center for Translational Cancer
    Research
Institute of Biosciences and
    Technology
Texas A&M Health Science Center
Houston, Texas

CONTRIBUTORS

Tim Eisen, BSc, MB BChir, PhD, FRCP
Professor of Medical Oncology
Department of Oncology
Cambridge Cancer Trials Centre
Cambridge, United Kingdom

M. Kay Garcia, DrPH, MSN, LAc
Acupuncturist
General Oncology
The University of Texas MD
    Anderson Cancer Center
Houston, Texas

Bishoy A. Gayed, MD
Assistant Instructor of Urology
University of Texas Southwestern
    Medical Center
Dallas, Texas

Amol J. Ghia, MD
Assistant Professor
Department of Radiation Oncology
The University of Texas MD
    Anderson Cancer Center
Houston, Texas

Jian Gu, PhD
Associate Professor
Department of Epidemiology
The University of Texas MD
    Anderson Cancer Center
Houston, Texas

Anasuya Gunturi, MD, PhD
Hematology/Oncology Fellow
Department of Medicine
Beth Israel Deaconess Medical
    Center
Boston, Massachusetts

Thai H. Ho, MD, PhD
Assistant Professor
Division of Hematology and
    Oncology
Mayo Clinic
Scottsdale, Arizona

Eric Jonasch, MD
Associate Professor of
    Genitourinary Medical Oncology
The University of Texas MD
    Anderson Cancer Center
Houston, Texas

Sarathi Kalra, MD
Postdoctoral Fellow
Department of Genitourinary
    Medical Oncology
The University of Texas MD
    Anderson Cancer Center
Houston, Texas

Jose A. Karam, MD
Assistant Professor of Urology
The University of Texas MD
    Anderson Cancer Center
Houston, Texas

Dae Y. Kim, MD, PhD
Urologic Oncology Fellow
Department of Urology
The University of Texas MD
    Anderson Cancer Center
Houston, Texas

Richard Lee, MD
Assistant Professor of Oncology
Medical Director of Integrative
    Medicine Center
The University of Texas MD
    Anderson Cancer Center
Houston, Texas

Gabriel Lopez, MD
Assistant Professor of Oncology
The University of Texas MD
    Anderson Cancer Center
Houston, Texas

Vitaly Margulis, MD
Assistant Professor of Urology
University of Texas Southwestern
    Medical Center
Dallas, Texas

xii

Surena F. Matin, MD, FACS
Professor of Urology
Division of Surgery
The University of Texas MD
    Anderson Cancer Center
Houston, Texas

David F. McDermott, MD
Associate Professor of Medicine
Harvard Medical School
Department of Hematology/
    Oncology
Beth Israel Deaconess Medical
    Center
Boston, Massachusetts

Sumanta K. Pal, MD
Assistant Professor
Department of Medical Oncology &
    Experimental Therapeutics
City of Hope Cancer Center
Duarte, California

George K. Philips, MB, BS
Associate Professor
Department of Oncology
Georgetown-Lombardi
    Comprehensive Cancer Center
Division of Hematology/Oncology
Medstar Georgetown University
    Hospital
Washington, DC

Priya Rao, MD
Assistant Professor of Pathology
Department of Pathology
The University of Texas MD
    Anderson Cancer Center
Houston, Texas

W. Kimryn Rathmell, MD, PhD
Associate Professor of Medicine
Division of Hematology and
    Oncology
University of North Carolina
Lineberger Cancer Center
Chapel Hill, North Carolina

Sharjeel H. Sabir, MD
Assistant Professor of Interventional
    Radiology
The University of Texas MD
    Anderson Cancer Center
Houston, Texas

**Ferdinandos Skoulidis, MD,
PhD, MRCP**
Academic Clinical Lecturer in
    Medical Oncology
Department of Oncology
University of Cambridge
Cambridge, United Kingdom

Xiang Shu, MS
Graduate Research Assistant
Department of Epidemiology
The University of Texas MD
    Anderson Cancer Center
Houston, Texas

**Alda L. Tam, MD, FRCPC,
MBA**
Assistant Professor of Diagnostic
    Radiology
The University of Texas MD
    Anderson Cancer Center
Houston, Texas

Pheroze Tamboli, MD
Professor of Pathology
The University of Texas MD
    Anderson Cancer Center
Houston, Texas

Cheryl L. Walker, PhD
Welch Chair and Director
Center for Translational Cancer
    Research
Institute of Biosciences and
    Technology
Texas A&M Health Science Center
Houston, Texas

Christopher G. Wood, MD, FACS

Professor and Deputy Chairman of
  Urology
The University of Texas MD
  Anderson Cancer Center
Houston, Texas

Xifeng Wu, MD, PhD

Professor and Department Chair of
  Epidemiology
The University of Texas MD
  Anderson Cancer Center
Houston, Texas

Sriram Yennurajalingam, MD, MS

Associate Professor of Medicine
Department of Palliative Care and
  Rehabilitation Medicine
University of Texas MD Anderson
  Cancer Center
Houston, Texas

Chapter 1

Epidemiology of Renal Cell Carcinoma

Xifeng Wu, Xiang Shu, Wong-Ho Chow, and Jian Gu

Introduction

The incidence rates of kidney cancer vary considerably worldwide, with much higher rates in North America, Europe, and Oceania than in Asia, South America, and Africa (Figure 1.1).[1] In the United States, kidney cancer is the sixth most common cancer in men and the eighth most common in women, with an estimated 65,150 new cases and 13,680 deaths in 2013.[2] The age-adjusted incidence rate in men (20.7 per 100,000 person-years) is nearly twice as high as in women (10.5 per 100,000 person-years). Likewise, the mortality rate for men (5.8 per 100,000 person-years) is double that of women (2.6 per 100,000 person-years).[3] The incidence rates of kidney cancer have steadily increased at more than 2% per year during the past three decades (Figure 1.1).[3] The rise in incidence has been more rapid in blacks than in whites. In contrast, mortality rates have been virtually identical for both blacks and whites since the early 1990s,[4] raising the possibility that the excess in kidney cancer incidence among black occurred largely in early-stage tumors with improved prognosis.

The etiology of renal cell carcinoma (RCC) differs from that of other kidney cancers. The remainder of this chapter focuses on RCC.

Several risk factors have been established for RCC, including obesity/being overweight, cigarette smoking, and hypertension. A few RCC susceptibility loci have been identified through recent genome-wide association studies (GWASs) of common single-nucleotide polymorphisms (SNPs). A number of intermediate phenotypic biomarkers in peripheral blood leukocytes (PBLs) have also been linked to RCC risk. In this chapter, we review the current state of knowledge on the epidemiology of RCC.

Modifiable Risk Factors

Cigarette Smoking

Cigarette smoking has been recognized as a causal risk factor with moderate effect on RCC. A large meta-analysis of 5 cohort and 19 case-control studies

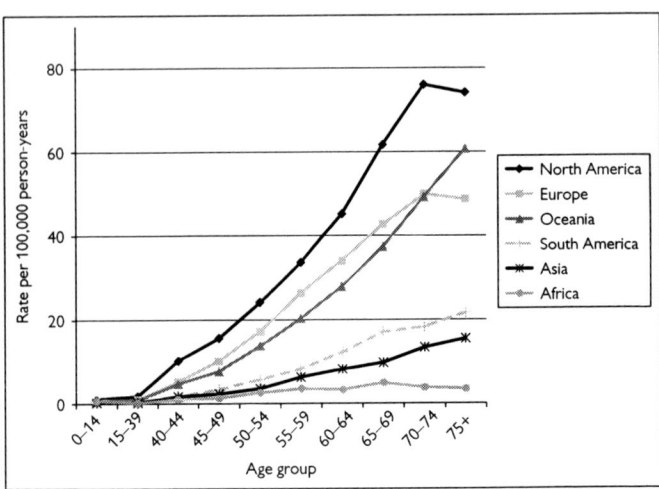

Figure 1.1 Worldwide estimated incidence rates of kidney cancer by age group. (Based on Ferlay J, et al. GLOBOCAN 2008.)

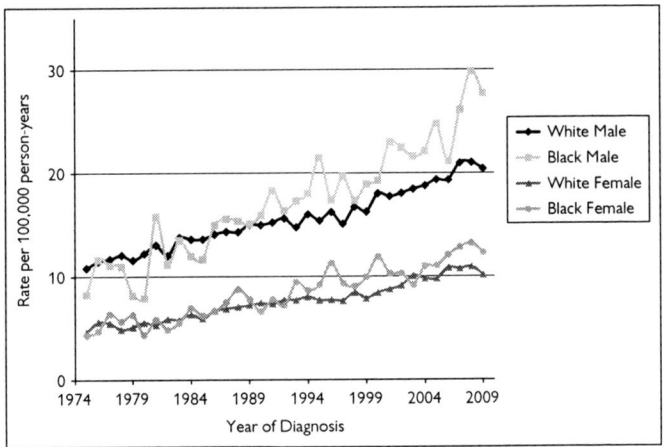

Figure 1.2 Trends in age-adjusted incidence of kidney cancer by race and sex, 1974–2009. (Based on nine areas: San Francisco, Connecticut, Detroit, Hawaii, Iowa, New Mexico, Seattle, Utah, and Atlanta.[3] The rate is age-adjusted to the 2000 US Standard Population.)

reported a 50% increase in RCC risk among male smokers and a 20% increase in risk among female smokers. RCC risk decreased by 15%–30% in both men and women who stopped smoking for more than 10 years.[5] Since the overall prevalence of cigarette smoking has declined for several decades in the

United States, smoking is unlikely to be a major contributor to the rising RCC incidence trends in this country.

A number of potential mechanisms that underlie the association between smoking and RCC have been proposed, including renal damage due to chronic tissue hypoxia caused by carbon monoxide exposure and smoking-related disorders such as chronic obstructive pulmonary disease, tubulotoxic effects, increased oxidative stress, and endothelial cell dysfunction.[6]

Hypertension

A meta-analysis of 18 studies showed a significant 1.6-fold increased risk of RCC associated with hypertension.[7] This association is independent of anti-hypertensive medications.[6] The biological mechanisms that relate hypertension to RCC are still unclear. Hypertension can induce chronic renal hypoxia and lipid peroxidation, and it is hypothesized that the resulting renal injury and metabolic or functional changes may subsequently increase renal susceptibility to carcinogens.

Obesity

In the United States about 40% of RCCs are estimated to be attributable to being overweight or obese.[4] Meta-analyses of prospective cohort studies showed that each 5-unit increase in body mass index (BMI) contributed an approximate 25%–35% increase in risk of RCC for men and women.[8] Weight gain during adulthood could be another risk factor for RCC independent of BMI per se, as reported in previous observational studies.[6] However, this association is still inconclusive due to conflicting results and confounding from obesity. Likewise, the effects of other related factors, such as weight cycling and waist–hip ratio, are also difficult to disentangle.

The potential mechanisms that underlie the association between obesity and RCC include altered production of circulating adipokines, insulin and insulin resistance, chronic tissue hypoxia, altered level of sex steroids, and lipid peroxidation and oxidative stress. Low levels of adiponectin have been associated with increased risks of RCC.[9] Hyperinsulinemia and insulin resistance have long been proposed as major mechanisms for the obesity–cancer link.[10] Chronic tissue hypoxia was supported by the frequent upregulation of hypoxia-inducible factor 1-α (HIF1-α) in RCC tumors.

Physical Activity

Physical activity has been associated with reduced RCC risks in a number of observational studies.[6] A cohort study showed that individuals who engaged in physical activity more than five times per week had a 20% reduction in RCC risk.[11] Two other cohort studies reported similar but statistically nonsignificant associations.[12,13] However, other cohort and case-control studies had null results.[6,14] The lack of consistent data may be partially attributed to the differences in measures of physical activity in the different studies, including leisure time physical activity during the past year, frequency of physical activity during a certain period, hours spent on physical activity per day or per week, and metabolic equivalent task values. Possible biological mechanisms for the beneficial effect of physical activity on RCC include reduced body weight/

BMI, improved insulin sensitivity, lowered blood pressure, and improved profile of inflammation and oxidative stress.

Diet and Alcohol Consumption

On average, one third of cancers are estimated to be attributable to diet and nutrition.[15] Daily diet is an important determinant of the amount of energy intake and is closely related to obesity. While dietary calorie intake may be associated with RCC risk, the effect is difficult to disentangle from BMI due to their tight correlation.

High fruit and vegetable consumption was associated with a >30% reduction of RCC risk in a pooled analysis of 13 cohort studies.[16] Intakes of fat and protein or their subtypes were not associated with RCC risk after adjusting for BMI, fruit and vegetable intake, and alcohol consumption in the same pooled analysis of cohort studies.[17] The reported associations of antioxidant nutrients including carotenoids and vitamins A, C, and E are inconsistent.[16,18,19] The intake of dietary acrylamide, which is concentrated in baked and fried carbohydrate-rich foods, was reported to confer a 60% increased risk of RCC in a case-cohort study in the Netherlands.[20]

Moderate alcohol consumption has been reported to be inversely associated with the risk of RCC.[21] A 28% reduction in risk was observed in people who consumed >15 g per day of alcohol, which is equivalent to one to two drinks per day; there was no further reduction with an additional increase in consumption.[22] A recent large prospective cohort study (a National Institutes of Health–American Association of Retired Persons diet and health study) found that alcohol consumption was inversely associated with RCC risk in a dose–response manner.[23] The associations with intake of other beverages, such as coffee, milk, and tea, are inconsistent.[6,24]

Other Medical, Occupational, and Environmental Factors

There are other reported risk factors for RCC, including type II diabetes mellitus, end-stage renal disease, long-term hemodialysis, acquired renal cystic disease, use of statins and aspirin, increasing parity and other reproductive factors, and occupational and other environmental exposures. However, the data are still inconclusive.[6,25]

Genetic Susceptibility

Hereditary Kidney Cancer Syndrome

Compelling evidence supports genetic susceptibility to RCC. The risk of RCC is two to three times higher in individuals who have first-degree relatives with kidney cancer.[26] In addition, familial aggregation is seen in approximately 3% of kidney cancer patients with inherited kidney cancer syndromes, which are discussed further in chapter 4.

Candidate Gene Approach

Most of the earlier candidate gene studies involved small numbers of cases and controls, and very few of the initially reported positive susceptibility alleles have been replicated in subsequent validation studies.[27] With regard to

RCC, candidate gene studies have reported many positive associations with SNPs in genes involved in xenobiotic metabolism, DNA repair, cell growth/apoptosis, inflammation, and other pathways.[6] None of the previously reported candidate SNPs have been replicated in large independent studies.

Genome-wide Association Studies

Two recent GWASs identified three novel genetic susceptibility loci mapped to 2p21, 11q13.3, and 12p11.23.[28,29] The observed effect size of each genetic locus is relatively small (odds ratio, 1.14–1.18), which is expected for common variants. Two validated SNPs are located in intron 1 of *EPAS1* (endothelial PAS domain-containing protein 1) on chromosome 2p21. *EPAS1* encodes *HIF-2α*, which is a biologically plausible causal gene in the von Hippel–Lindau-hypoxia-inducible factor (VHL-HIF) pathway. GWAS results provide further support for the involvement of *EPAS1* in RCC etiology.

The second interesting locus is mapped to *ITPR2* (inositol 1,4,5-trisphosphate receptor, type 2) on 12p11.23. Interestingly, the same SNP has also been identified as being associated with waist–hip ratio in another GWAS.[30] It is possible that obesity is the intermediate between the association of this locus and RCC. The third locus on 11q13.3 is mapped to an intergenic region with unknown biological function. Future pooled analysis of GWAS data will undoubtedly identify additional common RCC susceptibility SNPs.

Intermediate Phenotypic Assays for Renal Cell Carcinoma Susceptibility

Intermediate phenotypic biomarkers have the advantage of measuring the summary results of genetic variations and could potentially have larger effect size than individual SNPs. The suboptimal DNA damage/repair capacity in PBLs that were challenged with different mutagens has been shown to be associated with increased risks of RCC.[31–33] Shorter telomere in PBLs was associated with an increased risk of RCC.[34,35] Lower mitochondrial DNA (mtDNA) copy number in PBLs conferred an increased risk of RCC.[36] Prospective studies are needed to confirm these results from retrospective case-control studies.

Novel Biomarkers for Renal Cell Carcinoma Risk and Early Detection

Circulating microRNAs (miRNAs) are highly stable in a cell-free form protected from endogenous RNases and are promising biomarkers for cancer risk, diagnosis, and prognosis.[37] An earlier study of circulating miRNAs found an elevated level of miR-1233 in RCC patients.[38] Two recent studies also identified a few circulating miRNAs that were differentially detected in RCC patients compared with controls.[39,40] Metabolomics is an "omics" approach that is attracting tremendous interest in cancer research and biomarker discovery. Analyses of urine samples from RCC patients and control subjects have identified several potential biomarkers for diagnostics, including acyl-carnitine, quinolinate, 4-hydroxybenzoate, and gentisate.[41,42] For kidney and other urinary tract cancers, urinary markers may reflect the condition of the target organs directly and enhance the opportunity for discovery of promising diagnostic and prognostic markers specific to the urinary system.

Conclusions

The trend of increasing incidence rates of kidney cancer has been observed since the 1970s in the United States. The reason for this increase is not clear, although increasing rates of obesity and associated hypertension may partially explain this upward trend. Recent GWASs have identified three genetic susceptibility loci for RCC, and more common susceptibility SNPs are expected to be found from pooled analysis of GWASs. Next-generation sequencing is expected to provide significant biological insight into renal carcinogenesis. Prospective studies are needed for the discovery and validation of intermediate biomarkers. Additionally, the study of the gene–environment interaction in RCC etiology is an important next step. Finally, a comprehensive risk assessment model that integrates modifiable risk factors, genetic susceptibility loci, intermediate phenotypic biomarkers, circulating biomarkers, and gene–environment interaction is needed to move toward personalized risk assessment and cancer prevention.

References

1. Ferlay J, Shin HR, Bray F, et al. GLOBOCAN 2008 v2.0, Cancer Incidence and Mortality Worldwide: IARC CancerBase No. 10 [Internet]. Lyon, France: International Agency for Research on Cancer; 2010. Available from: http://globocan.iarc.fr.

2. Siegel R, Naishadham D, Jemal A. Cancer statistics, 2013. *CA Cancer J Clin.*. 2013;63(1):11–30.

3. Howlader N, Noone A, Krapcho M. SEER Cancer Statistics Review, 1975–2009 (Vintage 2009 Populations), National Cancer Institute. http://seer.cancer.gov/csr/1975_2009_pops09/. 2012.

4. Lipworth L, Tarone RE, McLaughlin JK. Renal cell cancer among African Americans: an epidemiologic review. *BMC Cancer.* 2011;11(133).

5. Hunt JD, van der Hel OL, McMillan GP, et al. Renal cell carcinoma in relation to cigarette smoking: meta-analysis of 24 studies. *Int J Cancer.* 2005;114(1):101–108.

6. Chow WH, Dong LM, Devesa SS. Epidemiology and risk factors for kidney cancer. *Nat Rev Urol.* 2010;7(5):245–257.

7. Corrao G, Scotti L, Bagnardi V, et al. Hypertension, antihypertensive therapy and renal-cell cancer: a meta-analysis. *Curr Drug Saf.* 2007;2(2):125–133.

8. Renehan AG, Tyson M, Egger M, et al. Body-mass index and incidence of cancer: a systematic review and meta-analysis of prospective observational studies. *Lancet.* 2008;371(9612):569–578.

9. Liao LM, Weinstein SJ, Pollak M, et al. Prediagnostic circulating adipokine concentrations and risk of renal cell carcinoma in male smokers. *Carcinogenesis.* 2013;34(1):109–112.

10. Calle EE, Kaaks R. Overweight, obesity and cancer: epidemiological evidence and proposed mechanisms. *Nat Rev Cancer.* 2004;4(8):579–591.

11. Moore SC, Chow WH, Schatzkin A, et al. Physical activity during adulthood and adolescence in relation to renal cell cancer. *Am J Epidemiol.* 2008;168(2):149–157.

12. van Dijk BA, Schouten LJ, Kiemeney LA, et al. Relation of height, body mass, energy intake, and physical activity to risk of renal cell carcinoma: results from the Netherlands Cohort Study. *Am J Epidemiol.* 2004;160(12):1159–1167.

13. Mahabir S, Leitzmann MF, Pietinen P, et al. Physical activity and renal cell cancer risk in a cohort of male smokers. *Int J Cancer.* 2004;108(4):600–605.

14. Bergstrom A, Terry P, Lindblad P, et al. Physical activity and risk of renal cell cancer. *Int J Cancer.* 2001;92(1):155–157.

15. Bingham S, Riboli E. Diet and cancer—the European Prospective Investigation into Cancer and Nutrition. *Nat Rev Cancer.* 2004;4(3):206–215.

16. Lee JE, Mannisto S, Spiegelman D, et al. Intakes of fruit, vegetables, and carotenoids and renal cell cancer risk: a pooled analysis of 13 prospective studies. *Cancer Epidemiol Biomarkers Prev.* 2009;18(6):1730–1739.

17. Lee JE, Spiegelman D, Hunter DJ, et al. Fat, protein, and meat consumption and renal cell cancer risk: a pooled analysis of 13 prospective studies. *J Natl Cancer Inst.* 2008;100(23):1695–1706.

18. van Dijk BA, Schouten LJ, Oosterwijk E, et al. Carotenoid and vitamin intake, von Hippel–Lindau gene mutations and sporadic renal cell carcinoma. *Cancer Causes Control.* 2008;19(2):125–134.

19. Lee JE, Giovannucci E, Smith-Warner SA, et al. Intakes of fruits, vegetables, vitamins A, C, and E, and carotenoids and risk of renal cell cancer. *Cancer Epidemiol Biomarkers Prev.* 2006;15(12):2445–2452.

20. Hogervorst JG, Schouten LJ, Konings EJ, et al. Dietary acrylamide intake and the risk of renal cell, bladder, and prostate cancer. *Am J Clin Nutr.* 2008;87(5):1428–1438.

21. Allen NE, Beral V, Casabonne D, et al. Moderate alcohol intake and cancer incidence in women. *J Natl Cancer Inst.* 2009;101(5):296–305.

22. Lee JE, Hunter DJ, Spiegelman D, et al. Alcohol intake and renal cell cancer in a pooled analysis of 12 prospective studies. *J Natl Cancer Inst.* 2007;99(10):801–810.

23. Lew JQ, Chow WH, Hollenbeck AR, et al. Alcohol consumption and risk of renal cell cancer: the NIH–AARP diet and health study. *Br J Cancer.* 2011;104(3):537–541.

24. Ljungberg B, Campbell SC, Choi HY, et al. The epidemiology of renal cell carcinoma. *Eur Urol.* 2011;60(4):615–621.

25. Chow WH, Devesa SS. Contemporary epidemiology of renal cell cancer. *Cancer J.* Sep- 2008;14(5):288–301.

26. Clague J, Lin J, Cassidy A, et al. Family history and risk of renal cell carcinoma: results from a case-control study and systematic meta-analysis. *Cancer Epidemiol Biomarkers Prev.* 2009;18(3):801–807.

27. Dong LM, Potter JD, White E, et al. Genetic susceptibility to cancer: the role of polymorphisms in candidate genes. *JAMA.* 2008;299(20):2423–2436.

28. Wu X, Scelo G, Purdue MP, et al. A genome-wide association study identifies a novel susceptibility locus for renal cell carcinoma on 12p11.23. *Hum Mol Genet.* 2012;21(2):456–462.

29. Purdue MP, Johansson M, Zelenika D, et al. Genome-wide association study of renal cell carcinoma identifies two susceptibility loci on 2p21 and 11q13.3. *Nat Genet.* 2011;43(1):60–65.

30. Heid IM, Jackson AU, Randall JC, et al. Meta-analysis identifies 13 new loci associated with waist–hip ratio and reveals sexual dimorphism in the genetic basis of fat distribution. *Nat Genet.* 2010;42(11):949–960.

31. Clague J, Shao L, Lin J, et al. Sensitivity to NNKOAc is associated with renal cancer risk. *Carcinogenesis.* 2009;30(4):706–710.

32. Lin X, Wood CG, Shao L, et al. Risk assessment of renal cell carcinoma using alkaline comet assay. *Cancer.* 2007;110(2):282–288.

33. Zhu Y, Horikawa Y, Yang H, et al. BPDE induced lymphocytic chromosome 3p deletions may predict renal cell carcinoma risk. *J Urol.* 2008;179(6):2416-2421.

34. Wentzensen IM, Mirabello L, Pfeiffer RM, et al. The association of telomere length and cancer: a meta-analysis. *Cancer Epidemiol Biomarkers Prev.* 2011;20(6):1238–1250.

35. Wu X, Amos CI, Zhu Y, et al. Telomere dysfunction: a potential cancer predisposition factor. *J Natl Cancer Inst.* 2003;95(16):1211–1218.

36. Xing J, Chen M, Wood CG, et al. Mitochondrial DNA content: its genetic heritability and association with renal cell carcinoma. *J Natl Cancer Inst.* 2008;100(15):1104–1112.

37. Mitchell PS, Parkin RK, Kroh EM, et al. Circulating microRNAs as stable blood-based markers for cancer detection. *Proc Natl Acad Sci U S A.* 2008;105(30):10513–10518.

38. Wulfken LM, Moritz R, Ohlmann C, et al. MicroRNAs in renal cell carcinoma: diagnostic implications of serum miR-1233 levels. *PLoS One.* 2011;6(9):e25787.

39. Redova M, Poprach A, Nekvindova J, et al. Circulating miR-378 and miR-451 in serum are potential biomarkers for renal cell carcinoma. *J Transl Med.* 2012;10:55.

40. Hauser S, Wulfken LM, Holdenrieder S, et al. Analysis of serum microRNAs (miR-26a-2*, miR-191, miR-337-3p and miR-378) as potential biomarkers in renal cell carcinoma. *Cancer Epidemiol.* 2012;36(4):391–394.

41. Kim K, Taylor SL, Ganti S, et al. Urine metabolomic analysis identifies potential biomarkers and pathogenic pathways in kidney cancer. *OMICS.* 2011;15(5):293–303.

42. Ganti S, Taylor SL, Kim K, et al. Urinary acylcarnitines are altered in human kidney cancer. *Int J Cancer.* 2012;130(12):2791–2800.

Chapter 2

Pathology of Renal Cell Carcinoma

Priya Rao and Pheroze Tamboli

Renal cell carcinoma (RCC) is a diverse group of malignant epithelial tumors of the kidney that vary in their natural history, biology, and morphologic appearance (both naked eye and light microscopic) and in their response to systemic therapy.

Renal Cell Carcinoma Classification

Over the past century there has been much iteration of classification systems for RCCs. The World Health Organization (WHO) developed the most current classification system (Table 2.1). This system was built on the foundations of two earlier works (the Heidelberg classification and the American Joint Committee on Cancer [AJCC] and the Union Internationale Contre le Cancer classification), both of which were published in 1997. Since the 2004 publication of the WHO classification, additional unique types of RCC have been reported (Table 2.1). Salient features of these tumors are listed in Table 2.2.

Clear-Cell Renal Cell Carcinoma

Clear-cell RCC (ccRCC) is the most common RCC type, representing 65%–75% of all RCCs reported in most series.[1,2] Most patients present with a solitary tumor; however, multiple synchronous tumors occur rarely. The typical ccRCC is a solid tumor with a bright yellow or light orange cut surface. Cyst formation, hemorrhage, and necrosis may be evident, depending on the tumor. Most ccRCCs are organ confined, while the rest are locally advanced with invasion into the perinephric adipose tissue, renal sinus adipose tissue, renal vein, or inferior vena cava. In some studies, the renal sinus has been identified as the main portal for the tumor to spread beyond the confines of the kidney. The presence of delicate, interconnecting, sinusoidal-type thin blood vessels is an important histologic feature seen on light microscopy. These blood vessels separate tumor cells into variable-size nests and tubules. The tumor cells usually have cells with clear cytoplasm, hence, the name *clear-cell* renal cell carcinoma, which is a result of accumulation of lipids and glycogen in the cell's cytoplasm. However, some tumor cells may have eosinophilic cytoplasm; the number of cells with eosinophilic cytoplasm varies

Table 2.1 Renal Cell Carcinoma Types

Renal Cell Carcinoma Types in the 2004 World Health Organization Classification

Clear-cell renal cell carcinoma

Multilocular clear-cell renal cell carcinoma

Papillary renal cell carcinoma

Chromophobe renal cell carcinoma

Carcinoma of the collecting ducts of Bellini

Renal medullary carcinoma

Xp11 translocation carcinoma

Mucinous tubular and spindle cell carcinoma

Carcinoma associated with neuroblastoma

Unclassified renal cell carcinoma

Newly Described Renal Cell Carcinoma Types

Tubulocystic renal cell carcinoma

Acquired cystic disease–associated renal cell carcinoma

Clear-cell papillary renal cell carcinoma

Primary thyroid-like follicular carcinoma

Hereditary leiomyomatosis-associated renal cell carcinoma

Succinate dehydrogenase–associated renal cell carcinoma

within individual tumors. Rare tumors maybe almost entirely composed of cells with eosinophilic cytoplasm. In some high-grade ccRCCs, tumor cells may have "rhabdoid" features, that is, single cells with large eccentrically placed nuclei and prominent eosinophilic cytoplasm. Considering the aforementioned, the morphologic diagnosis of ccRCC is not based solely the cell cytoplasm. Rather, the diagnosis is based on a combination of the pattern of cell growth, pattern of the vasculature, and the cytoplasmic characteristics of the tumor cells.

Papillary Renal Cell Carcinoma

Papillary renal cell carcinoma (PRCC) is the second most common RCC type, representing 10%–15% of all RCCs. PRCC is the tumor that is most often multifocal and bilateral and likely to metastasize to regional lymph nodes. Rarely, metastases to regional lymph nodes form a mass larger than the primary tumor in the kidney. These tumors are most often soft and friable, usually with abundant hemorrhage and necrosis. PRCCs that appear cystic on radiographic studies tend to have solid-appearing tumor at the periphery, while most of the center has tumor cells suspended in hemorrhagic fluid. Papilla formation is the typical morphologic feature; however, tumor cells may also form tubulopapillary forms and tubules; rarely, the papillae are so close together that they appear to form solid nests. Based on morphologic features, PRCC is further divided into type 1 and type 2.[3] Type 1 PRCCs have thin fibrovascular cores that are lined with a single layer of low cuboidal cells with scant pale cytoplasm and low nuclear-grade nuclei. Collections of foamy histiocytes and psammoma bodies (laminated calcifications) are more common

Table 2.2 Morphologic Features and Immunohistochemical Profile of Renal Cell Carcinoma Types

Renal Cell Carcinoma (RCC) Type	Morphologic Features	Immunohistochemical Profile
Clear RCC	Nests, sheets, or tubular architecture; thin-walled sinusoidal blood vessels; optically clear-cell cytoplasm	EMA, vimentin, RCC antigen, CD10, carbonic anhydrase IX positive; CK7, AMACR negative
Papillary RCC	Papillary, tubular, or solid architecture; frequent hemorrhage and necrosis; foamy macrophages and psammomatous microcalcifications	EMA, vimentin, RCC antigen, CK7, CD10, AMACR positive; type 2 tumors are frequently CK7 negative
	Type 1: Cuboidal cells with scant cytoplasm and small or inconspicuous nucleoli Type 2: Pseudostratified columnar cells with voluminous eosinophilic cytoplasm and prominent nucleoli	
Chromophobe RCC	Solid sheets, nests, or tubules; thick-walled blood vessels; clear to eosinophilic cytoplasm with prominent cell membranes; perinuclear clearing; wrinkled nuclear membrane	EMA, CK7, CD117 positive; vimetin, CD10, RCC antigen negative
Collecting duct RCC	Centrally located; glandular or tubulopapillary architecture; inflammatory and desmoplastic stroma; high-grade nuclei; dysplasia of adjacent collecting ducts	Ulex europeaus lectin, HMWCK, CK7, p63, vimentin positive; CD10, RCC antigen negative
Renal medullary carcinoma	Centrally located; tubulopapillary, reticular, or microcystic architecture; inflammatory and desmoplastic stroma with prominent neutrophilic infiltrate; high-grade nuclei; trepanocytes (sickled erythrocytes)	Ulex europeaus lectin, HMWCK, CK7, p63, vimentin positive; CD10, RCC antigen negative
Xp11 translocation carcinoma	Papillary and solid architecture; psammomatous microcalcifications; cells with voluminous clear to eosinophilic cytoplasm; eosinophilic cytoplasmic inclusions	TFE-3, CD10, AMACR positive; EMA, CK7, low-molecular-weight CK, HMWCK negative
Mucinous tubular and spindle cell carcinoma	Tubular and focally solid architecture; tubules lined with cuboidal cells; spindle cells with low-grade nuclei; mucinous extracellular matrix	EMA, vimentin, RCC antigen, CK7, CD10, AMACR positive
Clear-cell papillary RCC	Cystic and partly solid tumor; tubulopapillary architecture; clear cytoplasm; apically located, low-grade nuclei	CK7, EMA, vimentin positive; AMACR, CD10 negative

(Continued)

Table 2.2 (Continued)

Renal Cell Carcinoma (RCC) Type	Morphologic Features	Immunohistochemical Profile
Tubulocystic RCC	"Bubble-wrap" gross appearance; variably sized cysts embedded in fibrous stroma; clear to eosinophilic cytoplasm; prominent nucleoli	CK7, CD10, AMACR, vimentin positive; HMWCK negative
Primary thyroid-like follicular carcinoma	Tubular architecture; eosinophilic colloid-like material in lumen; grooved nuclei; nuclear pseudoinclusions	CK7, vimentin, PAX8 positive; TTF-1, thyroglobulin, RCC antigen negative

AMACR, alpha methyl acyl Co-racemase; CK, cytokeratin; EMA, epithelial membrane antigen; HMWCK, high-molecular-weight cytokeratin; RCC, renal cell carcinoma; TTF-1, thyroid transcription factor 1.

in type 1 PRCCs. Type 2 PRCCs have tall columnar pseudostratified cells with abundant eosinophilic cytoplasm and high-grade nuclei. At present, there are limited data that show differences in clinical outcomes and genetic abnormalities between type 1 and type 2 PRCCs.[3,4]

Chromophobe Renal Cell Carcinoma

Chromophobe renal cell carcinoma (ChRCC) is the third most common RCC type, yet accounts for only about 5% of all RCCs. First described in 1985, ChRCC has distinctive morphologic and genetic features that separate it from the other RCC types.[5,6] ChRCCs are soft solid tumors with a distinctive tan or tan–gray color. Microscopically, based on tinctorial properties of the cell cytoplasm, ChRCCs are divided into typical ChRCC and the eosinophilic variant. Tumor cells form sheets, nests, or broad alveoli, with interspersed thick-walled blood vessels (in contrast to the thin-walled vessels in ccRCC). Most ChRCCs have two types of cells—cells with clear cytoplasm and cells with eosinophilic cytoplasm, with one cell type predominating. Typical ChRCC predominantly has clear cells, while the eosinophilic variant is predominantly composed of eosinophilic cells. Clear cells have abundant cytoplasm with a frothy, flocculent, or bubbly appearance compared with the optically clear cytoplasm in ccRCC. Eosinophilic cells tend to be smaller with finely granular eosinophilic cytoplasm. In both cell types, cytoplasmic organelles are pushed to the cell periphery, forming a halo around the nucleus. Since the organelles are pushed to the periphery, cell membranes appear thick and prominent, superficially resembling plant cells. Tumor nuclei tend to be hyperchromatic, frequently binucleated, and usually have a wrinkled nuclear membrane. The perinuclear halo and wrinkled nuclei result in the cells looking like koilocytes.

Collecting Duct Carcinoma

Collecting duct carcinoma (CDC) is a rare, aggressive RCC that accounts for <1% of renal tumors. CDC arises from the renal medulla and is usually located in the central region of the kidney. Histologically, CDCs have a glandular or tubulopapillary growth pattern with high nuclear-grade cells that are associated with a prominent desmoplastic stromal response. Aggressive features such as necrosis, lymphovascular invasion, and high pathologic stage are common. Overall survival is poor.[7,8]

Renal Medullary Carcinoma

Renal medullary carcinoma (RMC) affects young adults with a history of sickle cell trait and is regarded as a sickle cell nephropathy.[9] Histologically, RMC resembles CDC with glandular, reticular, and microcystic features, occasionally having extracellular mucin. Most patients present with advanced disease, with a median survival of <1 year.[10]

Mucinous Tubular and Spindle Cell Carcinoma

Mucinous tubular and spindle cell carcinoma (MTSCC) is a rare RCC with distinctive morphology that overlaps with that of type 1 PRCC. As the name implies, these tumors are composed of tubules lined with cuboidal cells, extracellular mucin, and a bland spindle cell component. Most MTSCCs follow an indolent course when they are small and organ confined; however, larger tumors may be aggressive and possess sarcomatoid dedifferentiation.[8,11]

Renal Cell Carcinoma Associated with Xp11.2 Translocation

Xp11.2 translocation carcinoma is a distinctive RCC that is characterized by the presence of various translocations involving the TFE-3 gene located on chromosome Xp11.2, which is considered to be a part of the MiTF-TFE3 family of tumors.[12] While translocation RCC was first identified in a subset of pediatric RCCs, these tumors are now recognized as occurring in the adult population as well.[13] The two most common fusion partners to the TFE-3 gene are the PRCC gene t(X;1)(p11.2;q21) and the ASPL gene t(X;17)(p11.2;q25).[12] These RCCs have distinct morphologic features, with a papillary or nested architecture that often resembles a combination of ccRCC and PRCC. Tumor cells typically have abundant clear to eosinophilic cytoplasm, with some cells having prominent intracytoplasmic hyaline globules. Numerous psammomatous calcifications may be present. Demonstration of the translocation by fluorescence in situ hybridization or immunohistochemical detection of the nuclear TFE-3 protein is required for the diagnosis. These RCCs are generally aggressive, and patients often present with locally advanced disease.

Carcinoma Associated with Neuroblastoma

RCCs that are associated with neuroblastoma are rare tumors with distinctive histologic features that have been reported in pediatric patients who survived childhood neuroblastoma. Tumor cells typically have abundant eosinophilic or oncocytic cytoplasm.[14,15]

Unclassified Renal Cell Carcinoma

Unclassified RCC is a designation for RCC that does not fit into one of the known types and is not a distinct type by itself. Since 2004, new distinct RCC types have been reported (see section below). Unclassified RCCs also include tumors that are composites of known types, for example, ccRCC and PRCC, RCC with extensive necrosis and viable tumor that cannot be typed accurately, and RCC with sarcomatoid dedifferentiation in which the epithelial component cannot be readily assigned to one of the known RCC types.[16]

Sarcomatoid Dedifferentiation in Renal Cell Carcinoma

Approximately 1%–2% of RCCs undergo sarcomatoid dedifferentiation, which denotes transformation of the RCC into a high-grade biphasic tumor with both malignant epithelial (carcinoma) and mesenchymal (sarcoma) components. Sarcomatoid RCC was considered to be a distinct type of RCC; however, this term was discarded in the late 1990s, as all types of RCC may undergo dedifferentiation.[16] The carcinoma component may be any of the RCC types and is usually high grade but may be low grade. The sarcoma component is usually undifferentiated, resembling a pleomorphic malignant fibrous histiocytoma. Rarely, the sarcoma component shows heterologous differentiation into bone, cartilage, blood vessels, or muscle. Primary sarcomas of the kidney, which are rare, are included in the differential diagnosis. Finding a distinct carcinoma component helps separate primary renal sarcomas from RCCs with sarcomatoid dedifferentiation. Rarely, reactive spindle cells are present in RCCs, which should be distinguished from the sarcomatoid component. Most tumors have poor prognosis and present as high-stage tumors. The amount of tumor with sarcomatoid dedifferentiation (as a percentage of the entire tumor) has been reported to be prognostically significant. Patients who have RCCs with more than 50% sarcomatoid dedifferentiation tend to do poorly, but RCCs with even a minor sarcomatoid component (5%–15%) may result in metastasis and cancer-specific death.[17] However, newer data suggest a lack of correlation between percentage of sarcomatoid component and cancer-specific mortality.[18]

Newly Described Variants of Renal Cell Carcinoma

Since the 2004 WHO classification of RCC was published, there have been several newly described RCC types (Table 2.1), which are discussed below. In the past, tubulocystic RCC was erroneously referred to as low-grade CDC. The cut surfaces of these tumors have a characteristic "bubble-wrap" appearance, as they are composed of variable-size cysts set in a dense stroma. These cysts are lined with cells that have clear to eosinophilic cytoplasm, with a high Fuhrman nuclear grade (FNG; usually 3).[19]

Acquired cystic disease-associated RCC was first reported in 2006 in a series of patients with end-stage renal disease (ESRD).[20] These tumors occur exclusively in the setting of ESRD and have a strong association with dialysis. These tumors have characteristic microcystic architecture with eosinophilic tumor cells and high-grade nuclei. Calcium oxalate crystal deposits are a frequent pathologic finding. These tumors can occasionally be aggressive, and metastases have been reported.

Clear-cell papillary RCC (CCPRCC)was first described in the setting of ESRD but now has been reported to occur in the sporadic setting. Tumors are generally partially or extensively cystic, small, and organ confined. These tumors have delicate papillae lined with clear cells that have low-grade apically located nuclei. These tumors are indolent, and metastatic tumors have not been reported.[21]

Primary thyroid-like follicular carcinoma is histologically indistinguishable from follicular carcinoma of the thyroid gland and is composed of tubules with inspissated colloid-like material. Thyroid-specific immunohistochemical stains are negative, which helps with the diagnosis.[22]

Hereditary leiomyomatosis-associated RCC affects young patients with germline mutations of the fumarate hydratase gene. Patients may also develop cutaneous and uterine leiomyomas or leiomyosarcomas. Histologically, they resemble type2 PRCC with extensive tubulopapillary architecture, eosinophilic cells, and prominent orangeophilic "viral-like" nuclear inclusions. Patients usually present with locally advanced tumors, and prognosis is poor.[23]

Succinate dehydrogenase (SDH)-associated RCC is a recently described RCC type that is associated with germline mutations of the Krebs cycle enzyme, SDH, involving the SDH-B/C/D genes. The histology may be varied. SDH-B–associated RCCs frequently have an oncocytic appearance, while SDH-C–associated RCCs frequently show a clear-cell appearance. Patients often follow an aggressive clinical course.[24]

Pathologic Prognostic Factors

Pathologic factors that affect prognosis in RCC are briefly discussed below. Pathologic stage using the AJCC tumor, nodal, and metastasis (TNM) system is the most important factor in determining the patient's prognosis. Important changes in the TNM staging system include the inclusion of renal sinus invasion in the pT3a category (since 2002); the upstaging of direct invasion into the ipsilateral adrenal gland from pT3a to pT4 (since 2010); invasion of the renal vein, which was changed from pT3b to pT3a; and invasion into the inferior vena cava (changed from pT3c to pT3b).

FNG is used for grading RCC. It is based on nuclear size and nucleolar size to stratify tumors into four grades and is determined by the highest grade within the tumor and not the most predominant.[25] To date, use of FNG as a prognostic parameter has been validated only in ccRCC.[26]

Tumor necrosis is reported to be associated with poor prognosis and disease-specific death in patients with ccRCC and ChRCC, but not in patients withPRCC.[2,27]

RCC type is important as a prognostic factor, as some RCC types are more aggressive than others. Of the three most common types, ccRCC has the worst prognosis, followed by PRCC and then ChRCC.[2] Medullary RCC and CDC usually have the worst prognosis. RCC with sarcomatoid dedifferentiation has a worse prognosis than the same type of RCC without dedifferentiation.[28]

Other pathologic parameters associated with a poor outcome include the presence of lymphovascular invasion, renal sinus invasion, and sarcomatoid dedifferentiation.[28]

Ancillary Tests for Renal Cell Carcinoma Classification

Immunohistochemical stains are a useful adjunct in the diagnosis and work-up of RCC. Although the majority of RCCs are diagnosed without the use of ancillary techniques, immunohistochemical stains are useful in cases where morphology is not typical or in limited samples, for example, needle core biopsies and fine-needle aspiration biopsies. Most RCC tumors stain for cytokeratin (CK) cocktail and epithelial membrane antigen (EMA), except for translocation RCC, which may be negative. CK7 is a specialized cytokeratin stain that is expressed in PRCC, ChRCC, tubulocystic RCC, CCPRCC, and MTSCC; it is typically negative in ccRCC. High-molecular-weight CK34βE12 (HMWCK) and CK5/6 are positive in most CDCs. PAX gene proteins (PAX-2 and PAX-8) are expressed in most renal tumors and may be useful for identifying RCC in metastatic sites. However, these proteins are not specific as they are also expressed in primary tumors from other sites (such as ovary and thyroid).[29] Vimentin is an intermediate filament that is expressed in most mesenchymal tumors but in few carcinomas. All RCCs, with the exception of ChRCC, express this marker, which is useful for distinction between ccRCC and ChRCC. Alpha-methylacyl-CoA racemase (AMACR) is a mitochondrial enzyme that is involved in the oxidation of fatty acids and is strongly expressed in PRCC and MTSCC. While it may be expressed in other RCCs, the expression is typically focal and less strong than in PRCC and MTSCC.[29] CD10 is a cell surface glycoprotein that is typically expressed in ccRCC and PRCC, with less frequent expression in other RCCs.[29] RCC antigen is a glycoprotein that is present on the brush border of proximal renal tubular epithelial cells and is expressed in ccRCC and PRCC.[29] TFE-3/TFE-B are nuclear proteins that are overexpressed as a result of the specific translocation and accumulate in the nuclei of tumor cells in translocation RCC. These are highly specific markers and not expressed in any of the other RCCs.

Immunohistochemical profiles of the most common RCCs are as follows (Table 2.2): ccRCCs are positive for EMA, vimentin, RCC antigen, CD10, and carbonic anhydrase IX and negative for CK7 and AMACR. PRCCs and MTSCCs are positive for EMA, vimentin, RCC antigen, CK7, CD10, and AMACR. ChRCCs are positive for EMA, CK7, and CD117 and negative for vimetin, CD10, and RCC antigen. CDCs and medullary RCCs are positive for ulex europeaus lectin, HMWCK, CK7, p63, and vimentin and are negative for CD10 and RCC antigen. Xp11 translocation carcinomas are positive for TFE-3, CD10, and AMACR and negative for EMA, CK7, low-molecular-weight CK, and HMWCK.

Molecular testing for RCCs has not matured to the point of being part of the routine pathology evaluation.

References

1. Amin MB, Tamboli P, Javidan J, et al. Prognostic impact of histologic subtyping of adult renal epithelial neoplasms: an experience of 405 cases. *Am J Surg Pathol*. 2002;26(3):281–291.

2. Cheville JC, Lohse CM, Zincke H, Weaver AL, Blute ML. Comparisons of outcome and prognostic features among histologic subtypes of renal cell carcinoma. *Am J Surg Pathol*. 2003;27(5):612–624.

3. Delahunt B, Eble JN, McCredie MR, et al. Morphologic typing of papillary renal cell carcinoma: comparison of growth kinetics and patient survival in 66 cases. *Hum Pathol*. 2001;32(6):590–5.

4. Yang XJ, Tan MH, Kim HL, et al. A molecular classification of papillary renal cell carcinoma. *Cancer Res*. 2005;65(13):5628–5637.

5. Thoenes W, Storkel S, Rumpelt HJ, et al. Chromophobe cell renal carcinoma and its variants—a report on 32 cases. *J Pathol*. 1988;155(4):277–287.

6. Przybycin CG, Cronin AM, Darvishian F, et al. Chromophobe renal cell carcinoma: a clinicopathologic study of 203 tumors in 200 patients with primary resection at a single institution. *Am J Surg Pathol*. 2011;35(7):962–970.

7. Gupta R, Billis A, Shah RB, et al. Carcinoma of the collecting ducts of Bellini and renal medullary carcinoma: clinicopathologic analysis of 52 cases of rare aggressive subtypes of renal cell carcinoma with a focus on their interrelationship. *Am J Surg Pathol*. 2012;36(9):1265–1278.

8. Srigley JR, Delahunt B. Uncommon and recently described renal carcinomas. *Mod Pathol*. 2009;22(suppl 2):S2–23.

9. Davis CJ, Jr., Mostofi FK, Sesterhenn IA. Renal medullary carcinoma. The seventh sickle cell nephropathy. *Am J Surg Pathol*. 1995;19(1):1–11.

10. Rao P, Tannir NM, Tamboli P. Expression of OCT3/4 in renal medullary carcinoma represents a potential diagnostic pitfall. *Am J Surg Pathol*. 2012;36(4):583–588.

11. Dhillon J, Amin MB, Selbs E, et al. Mucinous tubular and spindle cell carcinoma of the kidney with sarcomatoid change. *Am J Surg Pathol*. 2009;33(1):44–49.

12. Argani P, Ladanyi M. Translocation carcinomas of the kidney. *Clin Lab Med*. 2005;25(2):363–378.

13. Choueiri TK, Lim ZD, Hirsch MS, et al. Vascular endothelial growth factor-targeted therapy for the treatment of adult metastatic Xp11.2 translocation renal cell carcinoma. *Cancer*. 2010;116(22):5219–5225.

14. Koyle MA, Hatch DA, Furness PD, 3rd, et al. Long-term urological complications in survivors younger than 15 months of advanced stage abdominal neuroblastoma. *J Urol*. 2001;166(4):1455–1458.

15. Medeiros LJ, Palmedo G, Krigman HR, Kovacs G, Beckwith JB. Oncocytoid renal cell carcinoma after neuroblastoma: a report of four cases of a distinct clinicopathologic entity. *Am J Surg Pathol*. 1999;23(7):772–780.

16. Storkel S, Eble JN, Adlakha K, et al. Classification of renal cell carcinoma: Workgroup No. 1. Union Internationale Contre le Cancer (UICC) and the American Joint Committee on Cancer (AJCC). *Cancer*. 1997;80(5):987–989.

17. de Peralta-Venturina M, Moch H, Amin M, et al. Sarcomatoid differentiation in renal cell carcinoma: a study of 101 cases. *Am J Surg Pathol*. 2001;25(3):275–284.

18. Shuch B, Said J, La Rochelle JC, et al. Cytoreductive nephrectomy for kidney cancer with sarcomatoid histology—is up-front resection indicated and, if not, is it avoidable? J Urol. 2009;182(5):2164–2171.

19. Amin MB, MacLennan GT, Gupta R, et al. Tubulocystic carcinoma of the kidney: clinicopathologic analysis of 31 cases of a distinctive rare subtype of renal cell carcinoma. Am J Surg Pathol. 2009;33(3):384–392.

20. Tickoo SK, dePeralta-Venturina MN, Harik LR, et al. Spectrum of epithelial neoplasms in end-stage renal disease: an experience from 66 tumor-bearing kidneys with emphasis on histologic patterns distinct from those in sporadic adult renal neoplasia. Am J Surg Pathol. 2006;30(2):141–153.

21. Aydin H, Chen L, Cheng L, et al. Clear cell tubulopapillary renal cell carcinoma: a study of 36 distinctive low-grade epithelial tumors of the kidney. Am J Surg Pathol. 2010;34(11):1608–1621.

22. Amin MB, Gupta R, Ondrej H, et al. Primary thyroid-like follicular carcinoma of the kidney: report of 6 cases of a histologically distinctive adult renal epithelial neoplasm. Am J Surg Pathol. 2009;33(3):393–400.

23. Merino MJ, Torres-Cabala C, Pinto P, Linehan WM. The morphologic spectrum of kidney tumors in hereditary leiomyomatosis and renal cell carcinoma (HLRCC) syndrome. Am J Surg Pathol. 2007;31(10):1578–1585.

24. Ricketts CJ, Shuch B, Vocke CD, et al. Succinate dehydrogenase kidney cancer: an aggressive example of the Warburg effect in cancer. J Urol. 2012;188(6):2063–2071.

25. Fuhrman SA, Lasky LC, Limas C. Prognostic significance of morphologic parameters in renal cell carcinoma. Am J Surg Pathol. 1982;6(7):655–663.

26. Lohse CM, Blute ML, Zincke H, Weaver AL, Cheville JC. Comparison of standardized and nonstandardized nuclear grade of renal cell carcinoma to predict outcome among 2,042 patients. Am J Clin Pathol. 2002;118(6):877–886.

27. Pichler M, Hutterer GC, Chromecki TF, et al. Histologic tumor necrosis is an independent prognostic indicator for clear cell and papillary renal cell carcinoma. Am J Clin Pathol. 2012;137(2):283–289.

28. Belsante M, Darwish O, Youssef R, et al. Lymphovascular invasion in clear cell renal cell carcinoma—association with disease-free and cancer-specific survival. Urol Oncol. 2014 Jan; 32(1):30, e23–28. doi: 10.1016/j.urolonc.2012.11.002. Epub 2013 Feb 18.

29. Shen SS, Truong LD, Scarpelli M, Lopez-Beltran A. Role of immunohistochemistry in diagnosing renal neoplasms: when is it really useful? Arch Pathol Lab Med. 2012;136(4):410–417.

Chapter 3

Biology of Renal Cell Carcinoma

Thai H. Ho, Ruhee Dere, and Cheryl L. Walker

Introduction

Counting both inherited and sporadic cases, renal cell carcinoma (RCC) is 1 of the top 10 leading causes of cancer death, affecting more than 50,000 patients annually. Surgery is often curative for early-stage tumors (I–III), with a 5-year overall survival rate of 59%–95%.[1] However, the median survival of patients with metastatic disease is approximately 2 years with systemic therapy. The most common histology is clear-cell renal cell carcinoma (ccRCC), and the molecular mechanism is linked to the inactivation of the von Hippel–Lindau tumor suppressor gene (*VHL*).[2] The *VHL* gene product, pVHL, acts as an oxygen sensor that regulates degradation of the hypoxia-inducible factor (HIF) transcription factor. HIF transactivates several target genes involved in cellular adaptation to hypoxia by binding hypoxia-related elements (HREs) to activate transcription of these targets, including vascular endothelial growth factor (VEGF). The mammalian target of rapamycin (mTOR) signaling cascade is often stimulated in ccRCC, and activation of the mTOR kinase pathway further augments HIF levels to subsequently activate HIF-dependent transcription.[3] The elucidation of VHL function and mTOR pathway activation served as a foundation for the discovery and approval of VEGF and mTOR inhibitors for RCC treatment. Secondary mutations recently identified in histone-modifying enzymes suggest that chromatin remodeling and alterations of histone modifications may play a role in RCC pathogenesis with distinct epigenetic phenotypes. This chapter summarizes the genetic mutations and aberrant signaling pathways that contribute to metastatic ccRCC.

von Hippel–Lindau Pathway

RCC is a diverse set of malignancies that originate from the renal parenchyma. In addition to ccRCC, other histologies include papillary, chromophobe, and translocation.[4] Rare subtypes include renal medullary and collecting duct. Hereditary familial syndromes with a predisposition for RCC have provided clues regarding the molecular pathogenesis of sporadic RCC. VHL disease is caused by germline mutations in the *VHL* gene that is located on chromosome

3p25.[2] VHL disease is characterized by an increased risk of ccRCC, pheochromocytomas, and hemangioblastomas.[5] Individuals affected by VHL disease inherit a nonfunctional *VHL* allele or have a *de novo* VHL mutation.[5] A stochastic secondary inactivation of the remaining allele leads to development of tumors (Figure 3.1). Similarly, in sporadic ccRCC, loss of heterozygosity at the *VHL* gene locus, somatic *VHL* mutations, or *VHL* hypermethylation leads to biallelic *VHL* inactivation.[6]

pVHL is the substrate recognition component of the ubiquitin ligase complex and directly binds to substrates such as the HIF transcription factor.[7] Oxygen levels regulate the interaction between pVHL and HIFα.[8] Recognition by pVHL requires the hydroxylation of HIFα on one of two conserved prolyl residues by oxygen-dependent enzymes within the EgIN family.[9] In normoxia, pVHL targets the HIFα subunit for polyubiquitination and proteasomal degradation.[10] pVHL suppresses the production of hypoxia-inducible mRNAs, including VEGF and erythropoietin.[11] Conversely, in hypoxic conditions or in pVHL-deficient or -mutant cells, HIFα binds to HIFβ to form a heterodimeric transcription factor that binds HREs in DNA in order to increase transcription of hypoxia-responsive genes.[12]

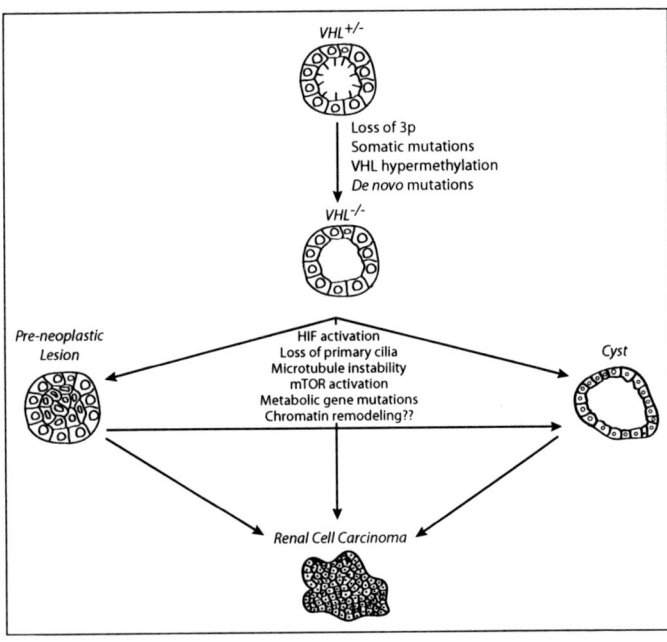

Figure 3.1 Biology of Renal Cell Carcinoma. Loss of 3p and *VHL* inactivation are likely early alterations compared to mutations in chromatin remodeling enzymes. Biallelic *VHL* inactivation drives HIF activation, and downstream signaling events that promotes tumorigenesis. Gene mutations that activate the mTOR pathway have also been characterized in both hereditary and sporadic forms of clear cell renal cell carcinoma. HIF indicates hypoxia-inducible factor; mTOR, mammalian target of rapamycin; *VHL*, von Hippel–Landau.

In addition to functioning as a key component of a ubiquitin ligase complex, pVHL has other cellular functions including maintaining the primary cilium. Loss of pVHL in ccRCC is associated with decreased cilia,[13] similar to what is observed in other ciliopathies such as polycystic kidney disease and tuberous sclerosis complex (TSC; Figure 3.1). Patients with mutations in genes associated with these ciliopathies display aberrant primary cilia, believed to result in multiple preneoplastic cysts.[14] Ectopic expression of VHL in pVHL-deficient RCC cell lines increases primary cilia formation.[15] The ciliary defect in VHL-deficient cells is attributed to elevated levels of aurora kinase A (AURKA),[16] a mitotic kinase that activates histone deacetylase 6 (HDAC-6) and disassembly of the cilium.[17] AURKA inhibitors have shown promise in vitro, and it is interesting to speculate on their benefit as preventative therapy to prevent cyst formation.

Mammalian Target of Rapamycin Pathway

The mTOR pathway responds to external and internal stimuli to regulate a diverse set of processes including cell proliferation, nutrient abundance, and protein synthesis.[18] mTOR acts as a scaffold for two distinct complexes: mTOR complex 1 (mTORC1) and mTOR complex 2 (mTORC2). The mTOR signaling cascade is under the tight regulation of tumor suppressors TSC2 (tuberin) and TSC1 (hamartin). These suppressors function as a heterodimer to act as a gatekeeper for this critical kinase. Activation of the PI3K-AKT-mTOR cascade results in the phosphorylation and inactivation of TSC2, which leads to derepression of mTORC1 inhibition.[19] Patients that inherit germline mutations in the *TSC1/2* genes are affected by hamartomas, renal angiomyolipomas, and RCC.[20] Loss-of-function mutations have been identified in *TSC1* in sporadic ccRCC that sensitize the VHL-deficient phenotype to mTOR inhibitors.[21] Rapalogs such as everolimus and temsirolimus inhibit mTORC1, but not mTORC2.[22] Dual inhibitors of mTORC1/2, currently in development, may provide additional benefit to rapalogs in RCC.[23]

Secondary Mutations of Chromatin Remodeling Genes in Clear-Cell Renal Cell Carcinoma

Although *VHL* is mutated in 65% of ccRCC, *Vhl* deletion in mice is insufficient for tumorigenesis.[1] Systematic sequencing of ccRCC identified loss-of-function mutations in histone-modifying enzymes such as *PBRM1* (41%), *BAP1* (15%), *SETD2* (3%), *KDM6A/UTX* (3%), *KDM5C/JARID1C* (3%), and *MLL2* (3%).[24–26] Eighty-eight percent of sequenced RCC with *SETD2* and *JARID1C* mutations also had *VHL* mutations, suggesting that these mutations may be modifiers of an RCC phenotype. Interestingly, several histone-modifying enzymes (*PBRM1*, *SETD2*, *BAP1*) reside on chromosome 3p where *VHL* is located. *PBRM1* encodes for baf180, a component of the polybromo BRG1-associated factor complex, which remodels the nucleosome to regulate transcription. Mutations in *PBRM1* are the second most common mutation after *VHL*.[25] Small interfering RNA–mediated depletion of PBRM1 expression in ccRCC cell lines resulted in both increased proliferation and cell migration.[25]

SETD2 was identified as a tumor suppressor in an insertional mutagenesis screen.[25] *Setd2* knockout is embryonically lethal in mice and has been shown to lack histone 3 lysine 36 tri-methylation (H3K36me3).[27] In a study examining the heterogeneity of mutations from random sampling within a RCC tumor, loss of function *SETD2* mutations were selected for in synchronous metastases.[28]

Exome sequencing identified truncating mutations in the C-terminal domain of *BAP1*, which encodes a H2A deubiquitinase.[26] Germline inheritance of *BAP1* mutations predisposes patients to mesotheliomas and melanomas.[29] Clinically, loss of BAP1 is associated with worse outcomes and more aggressive tumors.[30] Interestingly, in 70% of RCC cases, either BAP1 or PBRM1 are lost and are anticorrelated in expression, suggesting at least two distinct molecular epigenetic phenotypes.

Mutations in KDM5C/JARID1C, a H3K4me3 demethylase on the X chromosome, is associated with X-linked intellectual disability.[31] In RCC cell lines, hypoxia induces the expression of KDM5C/JARID1C in an HIF-dependent fashion to decrease H3K4me3 levels and alter gene expression.[32] Consistent with a tumor suppressor function, suppression of KDM5C/JARID1C increased tumor size in xenograft mouse models.[32]

Renal Cell Carcinoma as a Metabolic Disease

Hereditary leiomyomatosis and renal cell carcinoma (HLRCC) is a hereditary cancer syndrome characterized by cutaneous leiomyomata, uterine leiomyomas, and RCC.[33,34] Affected individuals inherit a germline mutation of fumarate hydratase (FH), a Krebs cycle enzyme (Figure 3.1). In HLRCC-associated RCC, both alleles are inactivated (germline and somatic), leading to a loss of FH.[34] Subsequent accumulation of the substrate, fumarate, inhibits prolyl hydroxylase, interferes with the recognition of HIFα by the pVHL, and leads to an increase in VEGF-mediated angiogenesis.[35] Succinate dehydrogenase-renal cell carcinoma (SDH-RCC), characterized by mutations of the Krebs cycle enzymes succinate dehydrogenase B or succinate dehydrogenase D, is associated with an increased disposition for pheochromocytomas and paragangliomas.[36] SDH mutations cause accumulation of succinate and inhibit prolyl hydroxylation of HIFα.[37]

Conclusions

The identification of additional mutations in genes other than *VHL* are changing our understanding of critical pathways that contribute to the development and progression of metastatic RCC (Figure 3.1). Drug targets may exist outside the mTOR and VEGF pathways, such as those aimed at the metabolic sensitivity or the tumor microenvironment in RCC. Mutations in "writers" of the genome that likely disrupt normal transcriptional regulation and chromatin remodeling will be crucial in increasing our understanding of the complex biology of RCC. In addition, the pleiotropic functions of pVHL have presented novel signaling cascades that are currently being dissected for their contributions to events that trigger tumorigenesis, including the loss of primary cilia and microtubule stability, with potential for preventative interventions. Thus, the identification of new "druggable" targets for sequential or combination therapies may provide a more robust form of therapy for RCC patients.

Bibliography

1. Cohen HT, McGovern FJ. Renal-cell carcinoma. *N Engl J Med.* 2005;353(23):2477–2490.

2. Latif F, Tory K, Gnarra J, et al. Identification of the von Hippel–Lindau disease tumor suppressor gene. *Science.* 1993;260(5112):1317–1320.

3. Barthelemy P, Hoch B, Chevreau C, et al. mTOR inhibitors in advanced renal cell carcinomas: from biology to clinical practice. *Crit Rev Oncol Hematol.* 2013; 88(1):42–56.

4. Storkel S, Eble JN, Adlakha K, et al. Classification of renal cell carcinoma: Workgroup No. 1. Union Internationale Contre le Cancer (UICC) and the American Joint Committee on Cancer (AJCC). *Cancer.* 1997;80(5):987–989.

5. Prowse AH, Webster AR, Richards FM, et al. Somatic inactivation of the VHL gene in Von Hippel–Lindau disease tumors. *Am J Hum Genet.* 1997;60(4):765–771.

6. Latif F, Duh FM, Gnarra J, et al. von Hippel–Lindau syndrome: cloning and identification of the plasma membrane Ca(++)-transporting ATPase isoform 2 gene that resides in the von Hippel–Lindau gene region. *Cancer Res.* 1993;53(4):861–867.

7. Cockman ME, Masson N, Mole DR, et al. Hypoxia inducible factor-alpha binding and ubiquitylation by the von Hippel–Lindau tumor suppressor protein. *J Biol Chem.* 2000;275(33):25733–25741.

8. Ivan M, Kondo K, Yang H, et al. HIFalpha targeted for VHL-mediated destruction by proline hydroxylation: implications for O2 sensing. *Science.* 2001;292 (5516):464–468.

9. Epstein AC, Gleadle JM, McNeill LA, et al. C. elegans EGL-9 and mammalian homologs define a family of dioxygenases that regulate HIF by prolyl hydroxylation. *Cell.* 2001;107(1):43–54.

10. Maxwell PH, Wiesener MS, Chang GW, et al. The tumour suppressor protein VHL targets hypoxia-inducible factors for oxygen-dependent proteolysis. *Nature.* 1999;399(6733):271–275.

11. Turner KJ, Moore JW, Jones A, et al. Expression of hypoxia-inducible factors in human renal cancer: relationship to angiogenesis and to the von Hippel–Lindau gene mutation. *Cancer Res.* 2002;62(10):2957–2961.

12. Semenza GL. Targeting HIF-1 for cancer therapy. *Nat Rev Cancer.* 2003;3(10):721–732.

13. Esteban MA, Harten SK, Tran MG, Maxwell PH. Formation of primary cilia in the renal epithelium is regulated by the von Hippel–Lindau tumor suppressor protein. *J Am Soc Nephrol.* 2006;17(7):1801–1806.

14. Hartman TR, Liu D, Zilfou JT, et al. The tuberous sclerosis proteins regulate formation of the primary cilium via a rapamycin-insensitive and polycystin 1-independent pathway. *Hum Mol Genet.* 2009;18(1):151–163.

15. Lutz MS, Burk RD. Primary cilium formation requires von Hippel–Lindau gene function in renal-derived cells. *Cancer Res.* 2006;66(14):6903–6907.

16. Xu J, Li H, Wang B, et al. VHL inactivation induces HEF1 and Aurora kinase A. *J Am Soc Nephrol.* 2010;21(12):2041–2046.

17. Pugacheva EN, Jablonski SA, Hartman TR, Henske EP, Golemis EA. HEF1-dependent Aurora A activation induces disassembly of the primary cilium. *Cell.* 2007;129(7):1351–1363.

18. Laplante M, Sabatini DM. mTOR signaling in growth control and disease. *Cell.* 2012;149(2):274–293.

19. Ma L, Chen Z, Erdjument-Bromage H, Tempst P, Pandolfi PP. Phosphorylation and functional inactivation of TSC2 by Erk implications for tuberous sclerosis and cancer pathogenesis. *Cell.* 2005;121(2):179–193.

20. Crino PB, Nathanson KL, Henske EP. The tuberous sclerosis complex. *N Engl J Med.* 2006;355(13):1345–1356.

21. Brugarolas J, Lei K, Hurley RL, et al. Regulation of mTOR function in response to hypoxia by REDD1 and the TSC1/TSC2 tumor suppressor complex. *Genes Dev.* 2004;18(23):2893–2904.

22. Thomas GV, Tran C, Mellinghoff IK, et al. Hypoxia-inducible factor determines sensitivity to inhibitors of mTOR in kidney cancer. *NatMed.* 006;12(1):122–127.

23. Chresta CM, Davies BR, Hickson I, et al. AZD8055 is a potent, selective, and orally bioavailable ATP-competitive mammalian target of rapamycin kinase inhibitor with in vitro and in vivo antitumor activity. *Cancer Res.* 2010;70(1):288–298.

24. Dalgliesh GL, Furge K, Greenman C, et al. Systematic sequencing of renal carcinoma reveals inactivation of histone modifying genes. *Nature.* 2010;463(7279):360–363.

25. Varela I, Tarpey P, Raine K, et al. Exome sequencing identifies frequent mutation of the SWI/SNF complex gene PBRM1 in renal carcinoma. *Nature.* 2011;469(7331):539–542.

26. Pena-Llopis S, Vega-Rubin-de-Celis S, Liao A, et al. BAP1 loss defines a new class of renal cell carcinoma. *Nat Genet.* 2012;44(7):751–759.

27. Hu M, Sun XJ, Zhang YL, et al. Histone H3 lysine 36 methyltransferase Hypb/Setd2 is required for embryonic vascular remodeling. *Proc Natl Acad Sci U S A.* 2010;107(7):2956–2961.

28. Gerlinger M, Rowan AJ, Horswell S, et al. Intratumor heterogeneity and branched evolution revealed by multiregion sequencing. *N EnglJMed.* 2012;366(10):883–892.

29. Carbone M, Yang H, Pass HI, Krausz T, Testa JR, Gaudino G. BAP1 and cancer. *Nat Rev Cancer.* 2013;13(3):153–159.

30. Kapur P, Pena-Llopis S, Christie A, et al. Effects on survival of BAP1 and PBRM1 mutations in sporadic clear-cell renal-cell carcinoma: a retrospective analysis with independent validation. *Lancet Oncol.* 2013;14(2):159–167.

31. Ounap K, Puusepp-Benazzouz H, Peters M, et al. A novel c.2T > C mutation of the KDM5C/JARID1C gene in one large family with X-linked intellectual disability. *Eur J Med Genet.* 2012;55(3):178–184.

32. Niu X, Zhang T, Liao L, et al. The von Hippel–Lindau tumor suppressor protein regulates gene expression and tumor growth through histone demethylase JARID1C. *Oncogene*. 2012;31(6):776–786.

33. Tomlinson IP, Alam NA, Rowan AJ, et al. Germline mutations in FH predispose to dominantly inherited uterine fibroids, skin leiomyomata and papillary renal cell cancer. *Nat Genet*. Apr 2002;30(4):406–10.

34. Toro JR, Nickerson ML, Wei MH, et al. Mutations in the fumarate hydratase gene cause hereditary leiomyomatosis and renal cell cancer in families in North America. *Am J Hum Genet*. 2003;73(1):95–106.

35. Kaelin WG Jr., Ratcliffe PJ. Oxygen sensing by metazoans: the central role of the HIF hydroxylase pathway. *MolCell*. 2008;30(4):393–402.

36. Ricketts CJ, Forman JR, Rattenberry E, et al. Tumor risks and genotype-phenotype-proteotype analysis in 358 patients with germline mutations in SDHB and SDHD. *Hum Mutat*. 2010;31(1):41–51.

37. MacKenzie ED, Selak MA, Tennant DA, et al. Cell-permeating alpha-ketoglutarate derivatives alleviate pseudohypoxia in succinate dehydrogenase-deficient cells. *Mol Cell Biol*. 2007;27(9):3282–3289.

Chapter 4

Inherited Renal Cell Carcinomas

Sarathi Kalra and Eric Jonasch

Introduction

Comprising only a small fraction of all renal tumors, inherited renal cell carcinomas (RCCs) have provided great insight into the molecular biology of RCC (Table 4.1). The first genetic evidence for the hereditary nature of RCC was from the discovery of the von Hippel–Lindau gene. Unlike sporadic cancers, inherited RCCs are usually bilateral and multiple and they develop at a younger age. Inherited variants having an increased risk for RCC include von Hippel–Lindau (VHL) disease, Birt–Hogg–Dubé (BHD) syndrome, hereditary papillary renal carcinoma (HPRC), hereditary leiomyomatosis and renal cell carcinoma (HLRCC), and tuberous sclerosis (TS).

von Hippel–Lindau Disease

VHL disease is an autosomal dominant disorder characterized by predisposition to a variety of benign and malignant tumors. The VHL spectrum comprises bilateral, multiple clear-cell kidney cancers; hemangioblastomas of the central nervous system (CNS); retinal capillary hemangioblastomas (RCH); pheochromocytomas; endolymphatic sac tumors of the middle ear; serous cystadenomas and neuroendocrine tumors of the pancreas; and papillary cystadenomas of the epididymis and broad ligament.

Epidemiology
VHL disease has an incidence of 1 in 36,000 live births. The disease manifestations can occur at any time of life, with a mean age at presentation of 26 years.[1]

Genetics
The *VHL* gene is a tumor suppressor gene. Although a germline mutation can inactivate one copy of the *VHL* gene in all the cells, the manifestations of VHL-associated tumors do not develop until the second "hit" prevents the expression of the remaining normal allele. The second hit can be through a somatic mutation, deletion, or hypermethylation of the promoter.[2]

Table 4.1 Hereditary Renal Cell Carcinoma Syndromes

Syndrome	Inheritance	Gene	Location	Pathway Involved	Genetic Testing Sensitivity (%)	Type	Phenotype
VHL	AD	VHL	3p25-26	–HIF-1	Nearly 100	Clear cell	Hemangioblastoma, pheochromocytoma, papillary cystadenoma, endolymphatic sac tumors of the middle ear, pancreatic cyst
BHD	AD with variable expressivity	BHD	17p11.2	mTOR	~88	Chromophobe, clear cell, papillary, oncocytoma	Fibrofolliculoma, trichodiscoma, acrochordon, and lung cysts
HPRC	AD	MET	7q31	HGF/MET	Unknown	Papillary type 1	None
HLRCC	AD	FH	1q42-43	Krebs cycle/HIF-1	~93	Papillary type 2	Skin and uterine leiomyomas
TS	AD with variable expressivity	TSC1 or TSC2	9q34 or 16p13	mTOR	Unknown	Clear cell, chromophobe, papillary, oncocytoma	CNS tumors, cardiac rhabdomyomas, angiofibromas of the skin

AD, autosomal dominant; BHD, Birt–Hogg–Dubé syndrome; CNS, central nervous system; HGF, hepatocyte growth factor; HIF, hypoxia-inducible factor; HLRCC, hereditary leiomyomatosis and renal cell carcinoma; HPRC, hereditary papillary renal carcinoma; MET, mesenchymal epithelial transition factor; mTOR, mammalian target of rapamycin; TS, tuberous sclerosis; TSC, tuberous sclerosis complex; VHL, von Hippel–Lindau disease.

Nearly 20% of patients with VHL disease have founder mutations, where the parents do not have a *VHL* germline mutation. Patients with founder mutations can be mosaics, that is, they express the mutation only in specific parts of their body. This feature may make detection of VHL disease more difficult, especially if the hematopoietic compartment is not affected, rendering blood germline testing useless.

The gene product is the 213 amino acid pVHL protein, which functions as a tumor suppressor. The pVHL protein binds with elongin B, elongin C, and cullin 2 to form a "VBC complex" and acts as an E3 ubiquitin ligase. This complex decreases intracellular protein levels of the transcription factors hypoxia-inducible factors-1α (HIF1-α) and HIF2-α via ubiquitin-mediated degradation. HIF in turn regulates the expression of a number of genes, including the proangiogenic vascular endothelial growth factor, platelet-derived growth factor-β, the glucose receptor GLUT1, and carbonic anhydrase IX. Loss of pVHL leads to an increase in HIF-α, even in a normoxic environment.[2]

Clinical Features

VHL disease has been classified into the following two major subtypes:

- Type I, which has a high risk of all tumors noted above except for pheochromocytoma, and
- Type II, which has pheochromocytoma with or without other neoplasms. It is further categorized as type IIA (without RCC), type IIB (with RCC), and type IIC (almost exclusively pheochromocytomas).

The majority of type 1 families have deletions or termination that lead to loss of VHL, whereas type 2 families are affected by missense mutations that reduce (but do not eliminate) the VHL function. The peak incidence of renal tumors is during the second and fourth decade of life.

VHL disease is the most common cause of hereditary RCC and comprises approximately 3% of the total RCC incidence. Patients with VHL disease are at risk for developing clear-cell RCC (ccRCC) and multiple renal cysts, which occur in nearly two thirds of VHL patients. The mean age of onset of RCC in VHL patients is 44 years, and nearly 70% of patients who survive to age 60 would have a tendency to develop RCC.[3]

The lesion most commonly associated with VHL disease is hemangioblastoma, affecting 60%–84% of patients. The majority of hemangioblastomas are located in the spinal cord, cerebellum, and brainstem, with only a small fraction of supratentorial lesions. VHL-associated hemangioblastomas tend to occur at younger age, with mean age of diagnosis of 29 years, whereas sporadic lesions occur one to two decades later.[1]

RCHs are also commonly seen in patients with VHL disease and will occur in up to 70% of VHL patients by age 60 years. RCHs are typically found either in the peripheral retina or the juxta-papillary region and are usually multifocal and bilateral. The mean age of presentation is 25 years.

The clinical criteria to diagnose VHL disease consist of a positive family history and one CNS hemangioblastoma, a pheochromocytoma, or a ccRCC. If there is no family history of VHL disease, then two or more CNS hemangioblastomas or one CNS hemangioblastoma and a visceral tumor (excluding epididymal or renal cysts) increase the suspicion toward VHL disease. Confirmation can be obtained by DNA sequencing and dosage analysis using multiplex ligation–dependent probe amplification or Southern blot analysis of the VHL gene. The sensitivity and specificity of these methods are nearly 100%.

Patients suspected of having VHL disease should be referred to specialized centers for evaluation, genetic counseling, and definitive diagnosis, even if there is no family history of VHL disease. Approved VHL clinical care centers are listed at http://www.vhl.org/patients-caregivers/living-with-vhl/clinical-care-centers/. These centers have been approved for standards of care that were developed by the VHL Family Alliance's Medical Advisory Board.

Medical therapy for VHL disease is experimental. Sunitinib has demonstrated a partial response rate by response evaluation criteria for solid tumors in RCC.[4] An ongoing clinical trial is testing pazopanib in the same patient population. In patients with hemangioblastoma, pazopanib has shown improvement of neurological signs and reduction in radiological tumor volume.[5] For RCC tumors larger than 3 cm, partial nephrectomy is the preferred surgical method and appears to be as effective as total nephrectomy.

Birt–Hogg–Dubé Syndrome

Drs. Birt, Hogg, and Dubé first described the autosomal dominant transmission of fibrofolliculomas with acrochordons and trichodiscomas. Later, BHD syndrome expanded to include extracutaneous manifestations such as pneumothorax, lung cysts, and renal tumors.

The BHD gene encodes for folliculin (FLCN), which is believed to act as a tumor suppressor. FLCN binds with two other proteins that bind to adenosine monophosphate–activated protein kinase. The complex that is formed eventually downregulates mammalian target of rapamycin (mTOR) activity.[6] Nearly 90% of the BHD mutations include insertion, deletion, somatic frameshift, or missense mutations. As a result, the truncated nonfunctional folliculin protein leads to increased activation of mTOR, which may contribute to RCC formation. RCC that is associated with BHD syndrome can present with a variety of histologies including (in decreasing order of frequency) chromophobe/oncocytic hybrid (nearly half of all the histological subtypes), chromophobe, clear-cell, oncocytoma, and papillary type.[7]

The renal manifestations of BHD syndrome remain clinically elusive, and the typical triad of hematuria, pain, and flank mass is only seen in a small fraction of patients. A path toward diagnosis begins with clinical suspicion, often raised by the discovery of suspicious cutaneous lesions that are confirmed by a dermatologist to be consistent with the stigmata of BHD syndrome. Radiological assessment usually includes computed tomography (CT) imaging, which helps in differentiating subtypes of RCC. Clear-cell, papillary, and collecting duct RCCs tend to show heterogeneous or peripheral enhancement, whereas chromophobe shows homogeneous enhancement with occasional calcifications.[8]

Genetic testing involves DNA-based diagnosis that consists of a sequence analysis and test for exonic deletions. Detection of an FLCN mutation confirms the diagnosis of BHD syndrome.

Chromophobe RCC has a better prognosis in comparison with other histological subtypes. The recurrence-free survival at 5 years for those who have had surgical resection is 83% and cancer-specific survival is 89%.

Hereditary Papillary Renal Carcinoma

HPRC is inherited in an autosomal dominant manner, where affected individuals are at risk of developing type 1 papillary RCC, which is bilateral and multifocal and associated with an early and late age of onset. Germline mutations occur in the *MET* proto-oncogene that encodes for MET, a transmembrane receptor tyrosine kinase. Hepatocyte growth factor binds to this receptor and acts in a paracrine manner to carry out various physiological processes including cell migration, proliferation, and tissue repair and regeneration. Although a number of different missense mutations have been identified, the majority of these lead to autophosphorylation of the MET protein, leading to overactivity and development of tumors.[9] Diagnosis is made by detecting the *MET* germline mutation, which may allow earlier diagnosis and treatment within families.

Hereditary Leiomyomatosis and Renal Cell Carcinoma

HLRCC is an autosomal dominant syndrome characterized by cutaneous and uterine leiomyomata and solitary, rapidly growing renal tumors with a papillary type 2 histology.[10] The renal tumors are highly aggressive and have a poor prognosis, warranting early detection in at-risk patients. Mutations in the *FH* gene are strongly associated with HLRCC. The *FH* gene encodes for fumarate hydratase, which converts fumarate to malate in the Krebs cycle. In the presence of a mutated FH protein, there is accumulation of fumarate, which inhibits the HIF-α prolyl-hydroxylase enzymes. This leads to accumulation of HIF-α in a fashion that is analogous to VHL mutations.[11]

HLRCC-associated renal tumors may cause hematuria, low back pain, and a palpable renal mass that is usually solitary and aggressive. Histologically, these renal tumors typically possess papillary features but can also demonstrate collecting duct or tubule papillary characteristics. The median age for detection of renal cancer in HLRCC is 44 years, and renal lesions occur in 10%–16% of all patients with HLRCC.

Clinical suspicion of HLRCC should be raised when there are multiple cutaneous leiomyomas with at least one histologically confirmed leiomyoma or a positive family history of HLRCC with one leiomyoma. Diagnosis is confirmed by testing FH enzyme activity in cultured skin fibroblasts or lymphoblastoid cells (which show a <60% activity) or by molecular genetic testing.[12]

Regular surveillance for skin lesions every 2 years, annual gynecologic evaluation, and an annual surveillance CT scan with contrast or magnetic resonance imaging for evaluation of renal lesions are imperative in at-risk individuals and family members of individuals diagnosed with the disease.

Tuberous Sclerosis

TS is an autosomal dominant condition in which affected individuals are at risk of developing multiple hamartomas in different organs. Only one third of TS cases are familial, whereas the remaining two-thirds can be due to spontaneous mutations or mosaicism. The following two genetic loci have been identified: one on chromosome 9 (*TSC1*) and one on chromosome 16p (*TSC2*) in a location immediately adjacent to the gene for the most common form of autosomal dominant polycystic kidney disease.[13] Renal lesions are seen in fewer than 5% of patients. Associated renal lesions are mainly angiomyolipomas (AMLs) that, despite their benign nature, can cause severe morbidity due to hemorrhage or compression of healthy renal tissue. CNS lesions cause the main clinical manifestations of TS, such as behavioral changes, epilepsy, and learning impairment.

The major issue with management of renal lesions in TS revolves around the potential of bleeding from AMLs. This can be managed by observation, surgical removal, and embolization (for tumors larger than 4–8 cm). Everolimus was Food and Drug Administration approved for the medical management of AMLs in 2012 based on phase II data showing clinical benefit in patients with TSC.

Translocation of Chromosome 3

A rare type of inherited RCC involves translocations from the short arm of chromosome 3 to chromosomes 2, 6, 8, or 11. The breaks in this variant are different from those seen in VHL disease, thus patients affected with this translocation do not develop manifestations similar to those of VHL disease (unless the VHL gene is involved in the translocation).

Akin to VHL patients, chromosome 3 translocation patients also have a tendency to develop ccRCC. The reasons for this unusual coincidence are not entirely understood. Studies suggest that the 3:8 translocation affects TRC8, which in turn may dysregulate p27 function in nascent tumor cells.[14,15] Further work is needed to understand the common elements in this rare RCC syndrome. VHL disease may provide insight into the steps required for the development of clear-cell kidney cancer.

Breast Cancer 1–Associated Protein-1 Mutation

Breast cancer 1 (BRCA1)–associated protein-1 (*BAP1*) is a tumor suppressor gene that encodes a nuclear deubiquitinase. *BAP1* germline mutations have been reported to be associated with uveal and cutaneous melanomas and mesotheliomas. Recently, a subset of ccRCC patients was reported to carry germline mutations in *BAP1*. *BAP1* inactivation was also seen in 15% of sporadic ccRCC cases and was associated with high Fuhrman grade and poor patient survival. *VHL* and *BAP1* are located on chromosome 3p. Several cases carrying *BAP1* mutations also showed *VHL* mutations, indicating that combined mutations may cooperate to foster ccRCC development or progression.[16]

Overview of Management of Hereditary Renal Cell Carcinoma Lesions

With the exception of VHL disease, no specific screening and surveillance guidelines have been laid out for hereditary cancers. Appropriate care for this patient group and their family members requires a blend of clinical suspicion, careful assessment of family history, and critical evaluation of the kidney on radiological imaging. Clinical evaluation should involve careful assessment for renal and extra-renal manifestations of the syndromes. Evaluation of the CNS, eyes, and cardiovascular system is essential in patients suspected of harboring VHL disease. Evaluation of the skin by a dermatologist and dermatopathologist is required for patients suspected of having BHD syndrome, HLRCC, or TS in order to rule in or rule out the presence of characteristic dermatological findings. The presence of cystic disease in the lungs of suspected BHD carriers can help to narrow down the diagnosis.

If a decision is made to perform genetic testing, the test should be performed under the supervision of a genetic counselor. Genetic counselors are equipped to address the psychological, social, legal, and biological consequences of a hereditary disease diagnosis and they can assist in the appropriate screening of additional at-risk family members.

When performing radiological assessment of the kidney, multiple cysts and enhancing tumors are suggestive of VHL disease; solid enhancing lesions in the absence of multiple cysts suggest BHD or HPRC syndrome; and large, solitary, and poorly enhancing lesions suggest HLRCC. Once the diagnosis has been made for the inherited RCC, it is important to analyze the causative germline mutation. However, these tests do not indicate the aggressiveness of the disease, hence imaging is a necessary modality to monitor the trends of growth of such lesions and also identify new lesions.

Usually, small tumors, especially those smaller than 3 cm, make partial nephrectomy a viable option. For VHL disease, HPRC, and BHD syndrome, tumors that are smaller than 3 cm in diameter generally are at low risk for metastasizing. Data on the behavior of renal masses of different sizes are lacking for other syndromes, and adopting the 3-cm guideline may be a reasonable approach if HLRCC is not suspected. For HLRCC, renal tumors tend to be aggressive, making it imperative to operate at the time of diagnosis, provided metastases have not occurred. Alternatives to partial nephrectomy include radiofrequency ablation and cryotherapy, which are most effective in tumors that are exophytic, located away from the hilum, and <4 cm in diameter.

Conclusion

The diagnosis of hereditary kidney cancer syndromes is important for the health of the affected individual as well as their family members. Timely screening of family members can lead to early detection and intervention for cancer and other organ manifestations associated with the syndrome, thereby decreasing disease-related morbidity for these individuals. Care must be taken to recognize the social, ethical, and legal concerns associated with a genetic diagnosis before disclosing the genetic information to family members, as the diagnosis affects the patient as well as their family members.

References

1. Lonser R, Glenn G, Walther M, et al. von Hippel–Lindau disease. *Lancet.* 2003;361(9374):2059–2067.

2. Kim WY, Kaelin WG. Role of VHL gene mutation in human cancer. *J Clin Oncol.* 2004;22(24):4991–5004.

3. Maher ER, Yates JR, Harries R, et al. Clinical features and natural history of von Hippel–Lindau disease. *Q J Med.* 1990;77(283):1151–1163.

4. Jonasch E, McCutcheon IE, Waguespack SG, et al. Pilot trial of sunitinib therapy in patients with von Hippel–Lindau disease. *Ann Oncol.* 2011;22(12):2 661–2666.

5. Kim BYS, Jonasch E, McCutcheon IE. Pazopanib therapy for cerebellar hemangioblastomas in von Hippel–Lindau disease: case report. *Target Oncol.* 2012;7(2):145–149.

6. Baba M, Hong S-B, Sharma N, et al. Folliculin encoded by the BHD gene interacts with a binding protein, FNIP1, and AMPK, and is involved in AMPK and mTOR signaling. *Proc Natl Acad Sci U S A.* 2006;103(42):15552–15557.

7. Pavlovich CP, Walther MM, Eyler RA, et al. Renal tumors in the Birt–Hogg–Dubé syndrome. *Am J Surg Pathol.* 2002;26(12):1542–1552.

8. Vera-Badillo FE, Conde E, Duran I. Chromophobe renal cell carcinoma: a review of an uncommon entity. *Int J Urol.* 2012;19(10):894–900.

9. Jeffers M, Schmidt L, Nakaigawa N, et al. Activating mutations for the met tyrosine kinase receptor in human cancer. *Proc Natl Acad Sci U S A.* 1997;94(21): 11445–11450.

10. Launonen V, Vierimaa O, Kiuru M, et al. Inherited susceptibility to uterine leiomyomas and renal cell cancer. *Proc Natl Acad Sci U S A.* 2001;98(6):3387–3392.

11. Sudarshan S, Linehan WM. Genetic basis of cancer of the kidney. *Semin Oncol.* 2006;33(5):544–551.

12. Pithukpakorn M, Wei M-H, Toure O, et al. Fumarate hydratase enzyme activity in lymphoblastoid cells and fibroblasts of individuals in families with hereditary leiomyomatosis and renal cell cancer. *J Med Genet.* 2006;43(9):755–62.

13. van Slegtenhorst M, de Hoogt R, Hermans C, et al. Identification of the tuberous sclerosis gene TSC1 on chromosome 9q34. *Science.* 1997;277(5327):805–808.

14. Gemmill RM, West JD, Boldog F, et al. The hereditary renal cell carcinoma 3;8 translocation fuses FHIT to a patched-related gene, TRC8. *Proc Natl Acad Sci U S A.* 1998;95(16):9572–9577.

15. Gemmill RM, Bemis LT, Lee JP, et al. The TRC8 hereditary kidney cancer gene suppresses growth and functions with VHL in a common pathway. *Oncogene*. 2002;21(22):3507–3516.

16. Farley MN, Schmidt LS, Mester JL, et al. A novel germline mutation in BAP1 predisposes to familial clear-cell renal cell carcinoma. *Mol Cancer Res*. 2013;11(9):1061–1071.

Chapter 5

Interventional Radiology Procedures in Renal Cell Carcinoma

Sharjeel H. Sabir and Alda L. Tam

Introduction

Interventional radiologists can be valuable members of a multidisciplinary treatment team. Team members can provide minimally invasive, image-guided diagnostic and therapeutic procedures for patients with renal cell carcinoma (RCC) such as image-guided biopsy, thermal ablation (TA), and transarterial embolization (TE).

Image-Guided Renal Mass Biopsy

Renal mass biopsy (RMB) is a procedure whereby a cannula is placed into the mass, through which smaller needles are placed to collect fine-needle aspirates and core biopsy specimens for cytopathological and histopathological analysis. Typically, computed tomographic (CT) or ultrasound is used to guide and confirm needle placement.

Renal masses are a common finding on diagnostic imaging, with 74% of new cases of RCC detected incidentally on imaging.[1] The probability of a renal mass representing RCC is correlated with the size of the mass: 72.1% measuring up to 2 cm, 75.1% between 2 cm and 2.9 cm, and 82.5% between 3 cm and 3.9 cm represent RCC.[1] The risk of metastases at presentation increases with tumor size, but patients with a 1-cm mass demonstrate a 1.4% synchronous metastasis rate.[2] Given this heterogeneous behavior of small renal masses (SRMs) measuring <4 cm, obtaining a definitive tissue diagnosis not only distinguishes between benign and malignant disease but also provides important prognostic information. Pathological analysis of a biopsy sample can establish the Fuhrman grade and histological subtype, both important prognostic factors.

Traditionally, SRMs were surgically excised without biopsy, which resulted in 17.3% of surgical resections being done for benign disease.[3] As smaller renal masses continue to be discovered,[4] a result of the increased use of cross-sectional imaging, the percentage of surgical resections for benign disease could increase. In addition, despite the earlier detection and surgical resection of RCC, there has not been a corresponding decline in mortality, calling into question current therapeutic algorithms[5] in which RMB does not play a prominent role. Thus, more recent management approaches have looked at incorporating RMB to guide treatment.[6]

The routine use of image-guided RMB, particularly in the management of SRMs, has been limited for several reasons. Based on studies performed before 2001, the false-negative rate of RMB was as high as 18% and the accuracy of RMB for cancer detection was as low as 88.9%.[7,8] However, in studies performed after 2001, the accuracy of RMB for cancer detection and determination of histological subtype is reported to be 96% and 94%, respectively.[7,8] The accuracy of RMB for assessing nuclear grade is 70%, which increases to 76%–100% if a simplified grading system (Fuhrman grade 1 and 2 are low risk and Fuhrman grade 3 and 4 are high risk) is used.[7,8] Another issue that has limited RMB is concern about complications, particularly track seeding. Modern techniques show a major complication rate of 0.3% and a minor complication rate of <5%.[7,8] The risk of tumor seeding is 0.01%, and no cases of track seeding have been reported when a coaxial cannula technique was used.[7,8]

Recent studies have shown the value of image-guided RMB for patients with SRMs. A 2013 study that used RMB as a basis for management decisions found that RMB guided appropriate therapy selection in up to 97% of patients.[6] Moreover, a recent cost-effectiveness analysis showed that use of RMB to determine whether patients should undergo surgery for an SRM would generally result in a similar life expectancy but at lower cost when compared with empiric surgery.[9] Lastly, in this era of personalized medicine, RMB provides a minimally invasive way to evaluate the genetic profile of an SRM, which could improve prognostication and guide management.[10]

Thermal Ablation

The most common percutaneous, image-guided TA techniques used to manage RCC are radiofrequency ablation (RFA) and cryoablation (CA). Other techniques such as high-intensity focused ultrasound and microwave ablation are not widely used, and studies are ongoing to determine their efficacy.[11,12]

Thermal Ablation for Primary Renal Cell Carcinoma
The increasing number of smaller RCCs being discovered has stimulated interest in nephron-sparing approaches for extirpation of these tumors. Partial nephrectomy is the standard of care for managing SRMs because of the lower occurrence of chronic kidney disease and equivalent oncologic outcomes when compared with radical nephrectomy.[13] However, for patients with SRMs where surgical options are limited, TA can play an important role.[14] For example, elderly patients, those with comorbidities that preclude surgery, patients with genetic syndromes that predispose them to multiple RCCs (Figure 5.1), and those with conditions that make nephron protection of the

highest importance are good candidates for TA.[14] The only absolute contra-indication to TA is an uncorrectable coagulopathy. Ideal lesions for TA are <4 cm, posteriorly located, and exophytic; however, larger tumors and those in other locations can be treated using techniques such as hydrodissection or pyeloperfusion in conjunction with TA, albeit with higher risks of incomplete ablation or complications.[15]

An advantage of TA over open partial nephrectomy (OPN) is the preservation of renal function. Patients with a solitary kidney who underwent OPN had a greater drop in estimated glomerular filtration rate compared with those patients who underwent RFA, 28.6% versus 11.4% ($P < 0.001$), respectively.[16] The overall effectiveness of TA for the treatment of primary RCC was addressed by a recent review that showed the overall recurrence-free survival for TA performed for SRM to be 84%–94%, with a cancer-specific

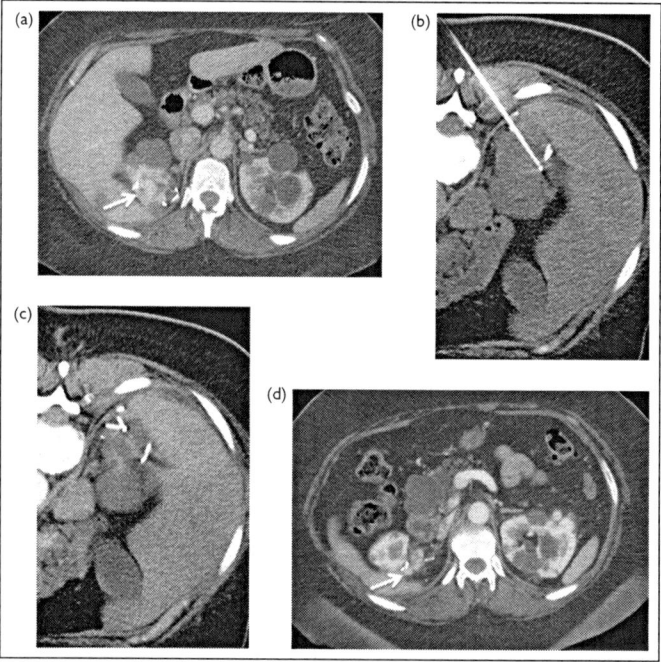

Figure 5.1 Radiofrequency ablation (RFA) used to treat a primary renal cell carcinoma (RCC) in a 46-year-old woman with von Hippel–Lindau disease. (A) Contrast-enhanced axial computed tomography (CT) demonstrates cysts within both kidneys and a small, solid, enhancing nodule (arrow) in the right kidney representing an RCC. Surgical clips are seen around the right kidney from a prior partial nephrectomy. (B) Noncontrast axial CT with the patient prone and an RFA probe in the RCC of the right kidney. (C) Post-ablation, contrast-enhanced axial CT showing no residual enhancement within the ablated RCC. (D) Contrast-enhanced axial CT obtained 2 years after RFA treatment shows involution of the ablation zone and no residual tumor (arrow). This CT showed development of a new enhancing nodule (not shown) in the contralateral kidney that was also treated with RFA.

survival of 89%–100%. No differences in the effectiveness or complication rate between percutaneous RFA and CA were found. Compared with laparoscopic TA, percutaneous TA was found to have a trend to fewer complications and decreased cost.[17]

Thermal Ablation for Metastatic Renal Cell Carcinoma

Cytoreductive nephrectomy and metastasectomy, both with demonstrated survival benefit,[18] remain important in the management of patients with metastatic RCC (mRCC). When surgery is not an option, percutaneous image-guided TA can be beneficial in select patients for addressing tumor in the kidney and metastases at various sites.

For instance, the survival benefit of kidney RFA as an alternative to cytoreductive nephrectomy in patients with mRCC who were not surgical candidates was shown in a small series of 15 patients.[19] In another study of 38 patients with mRCC who had 66 metastases to liver, lung, kidney, adrenal, and/or soft tissues, the overall survival during the average 10-month observation period was 100%.[20]

CA has also been used in the treatment of mRCC. Research is emerging that supports its use as a metastasectomy technique, particularly for musculoskeletal oligometastatic disease.[21]

Thermal Ablation for Palliation of Bone Pain from Metastatic Renal Cell Carcinoma

Osseous structures are the second most common site of metastatic disease in RCC after the lungs,[22] and 50% of patients who develop skeletal metastases from any primary cancer have poorly controlled pain during their disease course.[23] Because standard therapies (radiation, surgery, chemotherapy, and analgesics) have limitations, TA can be valuable in the management of bone pain (Figure 5.2). The mechanism for pain relief following TA is multifactorial and related to the destruction of sensory nerve fibers that supply the periosteum, debulking tumor volume, destruction of cytokine-producing tumor cells, and inhibition of osteoclast activity.[24]

Transarterial Embolization

During TE, a catheter is directed into the arteries that supply the tumor. Targeted delivery of an embolic agent is then performed with the intent of devascularizing the tumor and inducing necrosis. TE can be used as a tool for pain palliation, symptom control, and cytoreduction or as an adjunct to a planned surgical intervention. When preoperative embolization has been performed, surgical resection should follow within a 24- to 36-hour window in order to avoid revascularization.[25–27]

Embolization of Kidney Tumors

Preoperative TE of large renal masses has been evaluated for the reduction of intraoperative blood loss. In a group of 93 patients undergoing nephrectomy, 24 patients underwent preoperative renal artery embolization (RAE) with ethanol. In patients with renal masses >250 cc in volume (diameter of

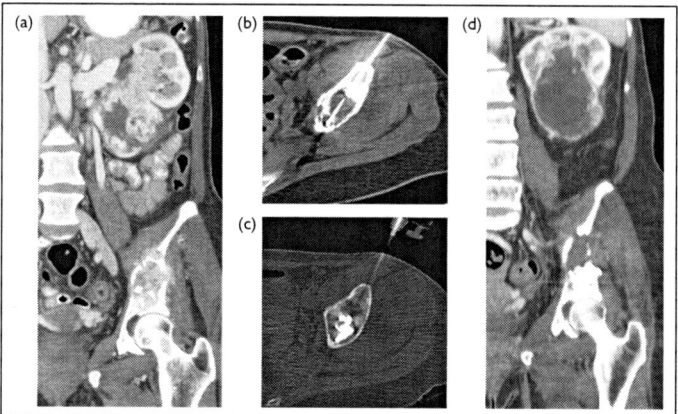

Figure 5.2 Cryoablation and cementoplasty used to palliate a painful left acetabular renal cell carcinoma (RCC) metastasis in a 57-year-old woman. (A) Baseline, contrast-enhanced, coronal computed tomography (CT) shows a bulky left renal mass and a large left acetabular metastasis with associated pathological fracture. (B) Axial CT showing placement of one of the four cryoablation probes used for cryoablation of the bone–soft tissue interface. (C) Axial CT shows placement of the polymethylmethacrylate cement on the day after cryoablation to stabilize the weight-bearing portion of the acetabulum. (D) Contrast-enhanced, coronal CT obtained 10 months after cryoablation shows no evidence of residual enhancing tumor in the acetabulum and no additional pathological fractures. The patient's pain was well controlled and she had started on pazopanib therapy, resulting in partial necrosis (absence of enhancement) of the left renal mass.

>7.4 cm) who underwent complete RAE, mean operative blood loss was significantly less than in those who did not undergo RAE (250 cc versus 800 cc; $P = 0.01$).[28] Whether preoperative RAE is associated with survival benefit is debatable, as one study demonstrated significant benefit[41] while another study of comparable design did not.[29]

TE of renal tumors can be used for cytoreduction. Of 54 patients with inoperable mRCC who underwent RAE with ethanol, the median survival was 229 days compared with 116 days for those in the control group ($P = 0.019$).[30] TE can also serve apalliative role by addressing specific symptoms such as hematuria (Figure 5.3),perinephric hematoma, flank pain, hypercalcemia, and hypertension.[31–33]

Embolization of Osseous Metastatic Disease

There are no prospective, randomized studies on the use of TE prior to resection of osseous metastases. However, retrospective data exist to document a significant reduction in intraoperative blood loss for mRCC patients who undergo preoperative embolization. For most surgeons, preoperative embolization is a prerequisite to spinal surgery.[34–41] TE can also be used as a technique for pain palliation from bone metastases. The devascularization and debulking of the tumor eases the compression and pressure effects on the periosteum, nerves, and surrounding structures to provide symptomatic relief.[42,43] The onset of pain relief can be as early as 12 hours following the procedure, and duration ranges from 2 to 12 months.[25,44]

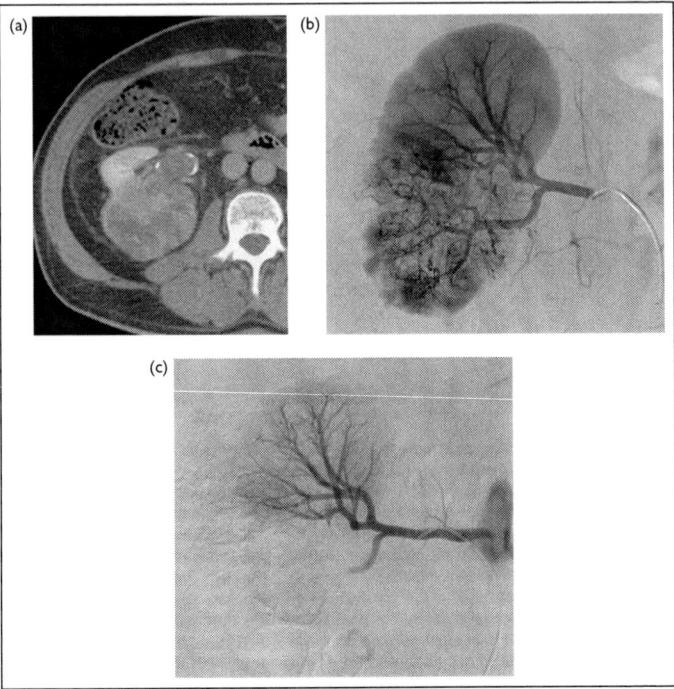

Figure 5.3 Transarterial embolization of a primary renal cell carcinoma with ethanol was done to palliate the symptoms of a 66-year-old man who developed gross hematuria after being placed on antiplatelet therapy following coronary artery stenting. (A) Contrast-enhanced axial computed tomography of the abdomen shows a 7-cm lower pole mass in the right kidney that invades the collecting system. (B) Pre-embolization digital subtraction angiogram (DSA) shows the hypervascular lower pole mass and its blood supply. (C) DSA after selective embolization of the inferior polar branch of the right renal artery with ethanol shows no further blood flow to the majority of the tumor. The patient's hematuria resolved after the procedure and he resumed antiplatelet therapy for his recently placed coronary artery stent.

References

1. Schlomer B, Figenshau RS, Yan Y, Venkatesh R, Bhayani SB. Pathological features of renal neoplasms classified by size and symptomatology. *J Urol.* 2006;176:1317–1320.

2. Nguyen MM, Gill IS. Effect of renal cancer size on the prevalence of metastasis at diagnosis and mortality. *J Urol.* 2009;181:1020–1027.

3. Pahernik S, Ziegler S, Roos F, Melchior SW, Thüroff JW. Small renal tumors: correlation of clinical and pathological features with tumor size. *J Urol.* 2007;178:414–417.

4. Nguyen MM, Gill IS, Ellison LM. The evolving presentation of renal carcinoma in the United States: trends from the Surveillance, Epidemiology, and End Results Program. *J Urol.* 2006;176:2397–2400.

5. Hollingsworth JM, Miller DC, Daignault S, Hollenbeck BK. Rising incidence of small renal masses: a need to reassess treatment effect. *J Natl Cancer Inst.* 2006;98:1331–1334.

6. Halverson SJ, Kunju LP, Bhalla R, et al. Accuracy of determining small renal mass management with risk stratified biopsies: confirmation by final pathology. *J Urol.* 2013;189:441–446.

7. Lane BR, Samplaski MK, Herts BR, Zhou M, Novick AC, Campbell SC. Renal mass biopsy—a renaissance? *J Urol.* 2008;179:20–27.

8. Samplaski MK, Zhou M, Lane BR, Herts B, Campbell SC. Renal mass sampling: an enlightened perspective. *Int J Urol.* 2011;18:5–19.

9. Pandharipande PV, Gervais DA, Hartman RI, et al. Renal mass biopsy to guide treatment decision for small incidental renal tumors: a cost-effectiveness analysis. *Radiology.* 2010;256:836–846.

10. Tan MH, Rogers CG, Cooper JT, et al. Gene expression profiling of renal cell carcinoma. *Clin Cancer Res.* 2004;10:6315S–6321S.

11. Carrafiello G, Mangini M, Fontana F, et al. Single-antenna microwave ablation under contrast-enhanced ultrasound guidance for treatment of small renal cell carcinoma: preliminary experience. *Cardiovasc Intervent Radiol.* 2010;33:367–374.

12. Klatte T, Marberger M. High-intensity focused ultrasound for the treatment of renal masses: current status and future potential. *Curr Opin Urol.* 2009;19:188–191.

13. Huang WC, Levey AS, Serio AM et al. Chronic kidney disease after nephrectomy in patients with renal cortical tumors: a retrospective cohort study. *Lancet Oncol.* 2006;7:735–740.

14. Campbell SC, Novick AC, Belldegrun A, et al. Guideline for management of the clinical T1 renal mass. *J Urol.* 2009;182:1271–1279.

15. Kumar AB, Trabulsi EJ, Lallas CD, Brown DB. Thermal ablation of renal cell carcinoma: triage, treatment, and follow-up. *J Vasc Interv Radiol.* 2010;21:S233–S241.

16. Raman JD, Raj GV, Lucas SM, et al. Renal functional outcomes for tumours in a solitary kidney managed by ablative or extirpative techniques. *BJU Int.* 2010;105:496–500.

17. Barwari K, de la Rosette JJ, Laguna MP. Focal therapy in renal cell carcinoma: which modality is best? *Eur Urol Supp.* 2011;10:e52–e57.

18. Breau RH, Blute ML. Surgery for renal cell carcinoma metastases. *Curr Opin Urol.* 2010;20:375–381.

19. Karam JA, Ahrar K, Wood CG, et al. Radiofrequency ablation of renal tumors in patients with metastatic renal cell carcinoma. *J Urol.* 2010;184:1882–1887.

20. Kloeters C, Mager AK, Johannsen M, et al. Radiofrequency ablation of metastases from renal cell carcinoma: technique, complications, and midterm outcome. *Eur Urol Supp.* 2007;6:653–657.

21. McMenomy BP, Kurup AN, Johnson GB, et al. Percutaneous cryoablation of musculoskeletal oligometastatic disease for complete remission. *J Vasc Interv Radiol.* 2013;24:207–213.

22. Motzer RJ, Bander NH, Nanus DM. Renal-cell carcinoma. *N Engl J Med.* 1996;335:865–875.

23. Callstrom MR, Dupuy DE, Solomon SB, et al. Percutaneous image-guided cryoablation of painful metastases involving bone. *Cancer.* 2013;119:1033–1041.

24. Callstrom MR, Charboneau JW, Goetz MP, et al. Painful metastases involving bone: feasibility of percutaneous CT- and US-guided radio-frequency ablation. *Radiology*. 2002;224:87–97.

25. Barton PP, Waneck RE, Karnel FJ, Ritschi P, Kramer J, Lechner GL. Embolization of bone metastases. *J Vasc Interv Radiol*. 1996;7:81–88.

26. Rowe DM, Becker GJ, Rabe FE, et al. Osseous metastases from renal cell carcinoma: embolization and surgery for restoration of function. Work in progress. *Radiology*. 1984;150:673–676.

27. Gellad FE, Sadato N, Numaguchi Y, Levine AM. Vascular metastatic lesions of the spine: preoperative embolization. *Radiology*. 1990;176:683–686.

28. Bakal CW, Cynamon J, Lakritz PS, Sprayregen S. Value of preoperative renal artery embolization in reducing blood transfusion requirements during nephrectomy for renal cell carcinoma. *J Vasc Interv Radiol*. 1993;4:727–731.

29. May M, Brookman-Amissah S, Pflanz S, Roigas J, Hoschke B, Kendel F. Pre-operative renal arterial embolisation does not provide survival benefit in patients with radical nephrectomy for renal cell carcinoma. *Br J Radiol*. 2009;82:724–731.

30. Onishi T, Oishi Y, Suzuki Y, et al. Prognostic evaluation of transcatheter arterial embolization for unresectable renal cell carcinoma with distant metastasis. *BJU Int*. 2001;87:312–315.

31. Maxwell NJ, Amer NS, Rogers E. Renal artery embolisation in the palliative treatment of renal carcinoma. *Br J Radiol*. 2007;80:96–102.

32. Munro NP, Woodhams S, Nawrocki JD, Fletcher MS, Thomas PJ. The role of transarterial embolization in the treatment of renal cell carcinoma. *BJU Int*. 2003;92:240–244.

33. Nurmi M, Satokari K, Puntala P. Renal artery embolization in the palliative treatment of renal adenocarcinoma. *Scan J Urol Nephrol*. 1987;21:93–96.

34. Chatziioannou AN, Johnson ME, Pneumaticos SG, Lawrence DD, Carrasco CH. Preoperative embolization of bone metastases from renal cell carcinoma. *Eur Radiol*. 2000;10:593–596.

35. Munke C, Bretschneider T, Lenhart M, et al. Spinal metastases from renal cell carcinoma: effect of preoperative particle embolization on intraoperative blood loss. *Am J Neuroradiol*. 2001;22:997–1003.

36. Breslau J, Eskridge JM. Preoperative embolization of spinal tumors. *J Vasc Interv Radiol*. 1995;6:871–875.

37. Smith TP, Gray L, Weinstein JN, Richardson WJ, Payne CS. Preoperative transarterial embolization of spinal column neoplasms. *J Vasc Interv Radiol*. 1995;6:863–869.

38. Olerud C, Jonsson H Jr., Lofberg AM, Lorelius LE, Sjostrom L. Embolization of spinal metastases reduces preoperative blood loss. 21 patients operated on for renal cell carcinoma. *Acta Orthop Scand*. 1993;64:9–12.

39. Berkefeld J, Scale D, Kirchner J, Heinrich T, Kollath J. Hypervascular spinal tumors: influence of the embolization technique on perioperative hemorrhage. *Am J Neuroradiol*. 1999;20:757–763.

40. Sundaresan N, Choi IS, Hughes JE, Sachdev VP, Berenstein A. Treatment of spinal metastases from kidney cancer by presurgical embolization and resection. *J Neurosurg*. 1990;73:548–554.

41. King GJ, Kostuik JP, McBroom RJ, Richardson W. Surgical management of metastatic renal carcinoma of the spine. *Spine*. 1991;16:265–271.

42. Chuang VP, Wallace S, Swanson D, et al. Arterial occlusion in the management of pain from metastatic renal carcinoma. *Radiology*. 1979;133:611–614.

43. Koike Y, Takizawa K, Ogawa Y, et al. Transcatheter arterial chemoemboliza- tion (TACE) or embolization (TAE) for symptomatic bone metastases as a palliative treatment. *Cardiovasc Intervent Radiol*. 2011;34:793–801.

44. Rossi G, Mavrogenis AF, Rimondi E, et al. Selective arterial embolisation for bone tumours: experience of 454 cases. *Radiol Med*. 2011;116:793–808.

Chapter 6

Management of Small Renal Masses and Early-Stage Renal Cell Carcinoma

Surena F. Matin

Introduction

With the increase in cross-sectional abdominal imaging modalities, the detection rate of small renal masses (SRMs), defined as measuring ≤4 cm in size, has increased from less than 15% of all renal masses diagnosed in the early 1970s to more than 50% in recent years.[1] Traditionally, radical nephrectomy was performed because most cases were identified at a higher stage and when the mass was of a larger size. With smaller tumors diagnosed at early stages, the goals of therapy are to achieve oncologic control and to preserve maximal renal function. In the management of SRMs, partial nephrectomy has become the reference-standard nephron-sparing therapy and has excellent long-term oncologic outcomes.[2] Parallel advances in surgical techniques have allowed radical and partial nephrectomy to be performed with minimally invasive techniques. However, for a subgroup of patients—those with competing morbidities, poor renal function, anatomic challenges, or hereditary syndromes, which make multiple interventions likely—surveillance and ablative therapies are potentially more attractive alternatives.

Active Surveillance

Surveillance of the SRM as an alternative to surgery was a novel concept when first introduced in 1995.[3] The context for greater acceptance for this option included a greater understanding of tumor biology, for example, the high incidence of benign tumors, particularly when tumors are smaller than 3 cm and patients are elderly, and the relationship between size and tumor progression that has been elaborated in patients with hereditary syndromes. Other factors that led to acceptance of surveillance were the recognition of competing risks of death and, worldwide, the threat of chronic kidney disease and its association with reduced survival. Surveillance represents the ultimate noninvasive, kidney-sparing option.

Several studies and metaanalyses assessing the outcomes of SRMs have been published in the past decade. Overall, these studies show a generally slow rate of growth, about 0.3 cm/year (a fast growth rate is generally accepted as >0.5 cm/year).[4] The risk of metastatic progression appears to be very low, and progression is generally seen in patients with tumors larger than 3 cm who are under observation.[5,6] Furthermore, delayed therapy does not seem to limit treatment options or confer a risk of stage progression.[4] It is also recognized that tumor growth does not provide evidence of malignant histology, as benign tumors have been documented to grow and renal cell carcinoma (RCC) may not.[5,7]

Candidates for surveillance include patients with SRMs <3 cm in diameter who are physiologically elderly and/or have significant medical comorbidities. Whenever possible, biopsy is encouraged in order to be proactively informed of the tumor's histology, particularly whether it is benign or malignant. Biopsy-proven benign tumors may be observed less stringently, for example, annually rather than semi-annually. However, since this type of tumor has been documented to grow, continued imaging is still recommended. The role of biopsy for active surveillance remains unclear. The common philosophy is that patients have a right to know whether they have cancer, even if it may not immediately alter management. With awareness of the nature of the mass, the physician can be more proactive if there are changes in tumor size over time. In some cases, patients may prefer to forgo biopsy since it may not alter management.

In regard to timing of surveillance, after two studies are obtained 3–4 months apart to establish the indolent nature of the lesion, imaging is performed every 6 months. In general, after 2 years, tumors that remain very indolent and with no change can be followed annually. Table 6.1 summarizes indications for surveillance and a suggested clinical pathway.

Thermal Ablation

Both cryoablation and radiofrequency ablation can be used in the kidney and are discussed in chapter 5. Indications and contraindications for ablative therapy are listed in Table 6.2.

Partial Nephrectomy

Several long-term studies have shown equivalent survival rates of patients who underwent nephron-sparing surgery (NSS) versus radical nephrectomy for a unilateral renal tumor <4 cm in size.[8–10] Rates of 5- and 10-year recurrence-free survival after NSS were shown to be comparable to those after radical nephrectomy. The risk of recurrence increases with larger tumors, bilateral tumors, multifocality, symptoms, and certain histologies such as papillary RCC.[11] Additionally, increasing attention should be given to the rising rates of chronic kidney disease, the interplay between kidney

Table 6.1 Indications and Suggested Clinical Pathway for Patients on Active Surveillance for a Small Renal Mass

Tumor Indications

Tumor diameter <3 cm (ideally)

Any tumor depth and location; these factors are relevant for consideration of biopsy only; small, completely intrarenal tumors have a high likelihood of nondiagnostic biopsy

Patient Indications

Elderly physiologic age or health status unfit for major surgery or anesthesia

Major medical comorbidities or another primary malignancy that requires active therapy

Need to minimize time off anticoagulation or antiplatelet compounds

Prior ipsilateral partial nephrectomy or other major renal surgery

Von Hippel–Lindau or other genetic syndrome

Chronic kidney disease

Contraindications

Relative contraindications:

-Young or healthy patient who is a candidate for definitive surgical extirpation

-Tumor >4 cm

-Hilar tumor location

Absolute contraindication:

-Uncontrolled coagulopathy

Suggested Clinical Pathway

Consider percutaneous core biopsy + fine-needle aspiration

Obtain second imaging study (if not already available) within 3–4 months to confirm that lesion is indolent

Obtain as first or second imaging a dedicated renal mass protocol computed tomography or magnetic resonance scan to confidently characterize mass; future imaging can be de-escalated if mass is well characterized initially

Continue imaging every 6 months

After 2 years, if mass remains unchanged and <2 cm in the setting of elderly age, consider following annually

---

disease and cardiovascular disease, and the association of subsequent kidney disease with radical nephrectomy. A European randomized study of partial versus radical nephrectomy has raised some questions regarding the benefit of NSS.[12] However, given the contradictory results within the study and the small numbers of patients that resulted in early termination, the shift toward favoring NSS continues.

Contemporary indications for NSS are listed in Table 6.3. Recent prospective data suggest a significant improvement in quality of life for patients who undergo NSS versus radical nephrectomy.[13–15] However, there remains some question regarding those who undergo radical nephrectomy and have less worry, while those with better renal function enjoy a better quality of life.[16] Patients who undergo NSS appear to have a lower long-term risk of renal failure.[17]

Table 6.2 Indications and Contraindications for Ablative Therapy

Tumor Indications

Tumor diameter <3.5 cm (ideally)

Enlargement of renal mass to ≥3 cm during active surveillance

Peripheral location; a central location is less favorable but not a contraindication

Tumor location appropriate for percutaneous or laparoscopic access
- Lower pole tumors at higher risk for ureteral injury during percutaneous route
- Anterior tumors near bowel not ideal for percutaneous route without adjunctive maneuvers

Patient Indications

Elderly physiologic age or health status unfit for major surgery

Major medical comorbidities or another primary malignancy that requires active therapy

Von Hippel–Lindau or other genetic syndrome

Chronic kidney disease

Solitary kidney

Prior partial nephrectomy

Contraindications

Young or healthy patient who is a candidate for definitive surgical extirpation

Uncontrolled coagulopathy

Table 6.3 Indications, Considerations, and Contraindications for Nephron-Sparing Surgery

Tumor Indications

Single renal tumor <4 cm, normal contralateral kidney

Single polar tumor 4–7 cm, normal contralateral kidney

Any size tumor with any of the following:
- Bilateral renal tumors
- Systemic condition that threatens renal function (eg, diabetes mellitus)
- Local condition that threatens contralateral kidney (eg, stone disease, renal artery stenosis)
- Chronic kidney disease
- Solitary functioning kidney

Considerations

Be mindful that central and hilar tumors have higher risk of hemorrhage and urinary leakage but are not contraindicated for partial nephrectomy

Minimize ischemia time to maintain long-term renal function

Resect minimal surrounding normal renal tissue

Contraindications

Uncontrolled coagulopathy

Radical Nephrectomy

Radical nephrectomy was considered the gold standard for kidney cancer for many decades until it was recently supplanted by partial nephrectomy. Fifty years ago the original description of radical nephrectomy included early vascular ligation, extrafascial dissection of the kidney outside Gerota's fascia, en bloc resection of the adrenal gland, and extensive lymphadenectomy from the crus of the diaphragm to the aortic bifurcation.[18–20] Since then, we have learned that such "radical" maneuvers are largely unnecessary, including routine removal of the ipsilateral adrenal gland and extensive lymphadenectomy, the role of which remains controversial from a therapeutic perspective.[21,22] Additionally, the open radical nephrectomy approach has been largely supplanted by a laparoscopic one, particularly for low to intermediate clinical-stage primary tumors, as described in the next section. In general, in contemporary practice, an open radical nephrectomy for treatment of a cT1a RCC would be considered not only overly invasive but also overextirpative from a surgical standpoint. Similarly, a laparoscopic radical nephrectomy (LRN) for a cT1a RCC, in general, would appear to be overtreatment. Certainly, individual patient and tumor factors, anticipated morbidity, and anticipated post-operative renal function play a role in shared decision-making discussions with the patient.

Laparoscopic and Robotic Approaches

Several 5- and 10-year follow-up studies have shown equivalent survival of patients who underwent LRN versus open radical nephrectomy.[23,24] The well-documented benefits of LRN include reduced blood loss, reduced pain and narcotic analgesic requirement, quicker ambulation, faster resumption of oral diet, shorter hospitalization, and more rapid convalescence. Table 6.4 summarizes contemporary indications for an LRN. Owing to continued advances in technology and surgical innovation, it is expected that some of these indications may be conducive to less invasive approaches. Most clinical T1-2 tumors <13 cm in size and some T3a-b tumors are amenable to laparoscopic excision.[23–25] Complication rates are comparable to those for open surgery, with an overall average of approximately 12%–15%.[25–27] LRN is an accepted standard for the overwhelming majority of clinically localized RCCs and for some locally advanced cases. Laparoscopic cytoreductive nephrectomy for patients with metastatic disease is associated with the same advantages as in the nonmetastatic setting and, as a result of the more rapid recovery, may be associated with a shorter time until initiation of systemic therapy.[28,29]

More recently, disturbing trends have been noted in regard to the overuse of radical nephrectomy for SRMs that could otherwise be treated by partial nephrectomy.[30,31] It appears that owing to the ease of performing a laparoscopic nephrectomy and its dissemination, coupled with slow acceptance of partial nephrectomy and the more difficult training for minimally invasive partial nephrectomy, most urologists are opting for minimally invasive complete

Table 6.4 Indications and Contraindications for Laparoscopic Radical Nephrectomy

Indications
Tumor diameter >4 cm; <13 cm (upper limit based on surgeon assessment)
Clinical stage T1, T2, T3a (perinephric or sinus extension)
M+ disease fulfilling above criteria, with good performance status
Contraindications
Relative contraindications (dependent on surgeon and individual findings): - Extensive perinephric extension - Prior renal surgery - Tumor amenable to partial nephrectomy - Hilar adenopathy - Tumor thrombus within vena cava (cT3a-c) - Invasion of surrounding organs (cT4)
Absolute contraindications: - Uncontrolled coagulopathy

removal. This comes at a time when we are more acutely aware of long-term dangers and concerns regarding chronic kidney disease.[32] It is hoped that the introduction of robotic laparoscopic approaches will increase the use of minimally invasive partial nephrectomy.

When performed by high-volume urologists, LPN has been shown to be an effective, minimally invasive nephron-sparing approach for selected small renal tumors.[33] It largely adheres to principles of open surgery, including hilar clamping, sharp dissection of the renal tumor with a margin of normal tissue in a bloodless field, suture ligation of the pelvicalyceal collecting system and central renal vessels, and parenchymal reconstruction.[33] However, it remains a challenging surgical endeavor that requires extensive laparoscopic experience. With the advent of a robotic surgery platform (eg, daVinci, Intuitive Corp., Sunnyvale, CA), which enables and facilitates laparoscopic surgery, the laparoscopic approach to NSS may be facilitated.

Robotic partial nephrectomy (RPN) represents the most recent evolution of minimally invasive NSS. Given the concern about overuse of LRN, the growing popularity of RPN may enable a larger number of urologists to provide minimally invasive NSS to their patients. Current data suggest that RPN is associated with a shorter warm ischemia time and a shorter operation than LPN, with these advantages being seen even for surgeons experienced with LPN.[34,35]

References

1. Fisher HA. Management of small renal cancers: choices for the patient and physician. *J Urol.* 2006;176(5):1907–1908.

2. Campbell SC, Novick AC, Belldegrun A, et al. Guideline for management of the clinical T1 renal mass. *J Urol.* 2009;182(4):1271–1279.

3. Bosniak MA. Observation of small incidentally detected renal masses. *Semin Urol Oncol.* 1995;13:267–272.

4. Kunkle DA, Egleston BL, Uzzo RG. Excise, ablate or observe: the small renal mass dilemma—a meta-analysis and review. *J Urol.* 2008;179(4):1227–1233.

5. Kunkle DA, Crispen PL, Chen DYT, Greenberg RE, Uzzo RG. Enhancing renal masses with zero net growth during active surveillance. *J Urol.* 2007;177(3):849–853.

6. Kunkle DA, Crispen PL, Li T, Uzzo RG. Tumor size predicts synchronous metastatic renal cell carcinoma: implications for surveillance of small renal masses. *J Urol.* 2007;177(5):1692–1696; discussion 1697.

7. Kawaguchi S, Fernandes KA, Finelli A, Robinette M, Fleshner N, Jewett MA. Most renal oncocytomas appear to grow: observations of tumor kinetics with active surveillance. *J Urol.* 2011;186(4):1218–1222.

8. Novick AC, Gephardt G, Guz B, Steinmuller D, Tubbs RR. Long-term follow-up after partial removal of a solitary kidney [see comments]. *N Engl J Med.* 1991;325(15):1058–1062.

9. Belldegrun A, Tsui KH, deKernion JB, Smith RB. Efficacy of nephron-sparing surgery for renal cell carcinoma: analysis based on the new 1997 tumor-node-metastasis staging system. *J Clin Oncol.* 1999;17(9):2868–2875.

10. Herr HW. Partial nephrectomy for unilateral renal carcinoma and a normal contralateral kidney: 10-year followup. *J Urol.* 1999;161(1):33–34; discussion 34–35.

11. Fergany AF, Hafez KS, Novick AC. Long-term results of nephron sparing surgery for localized renal cell carcinoma: 10-year followup. *J Urol.* 2000;163(2):442–445.

12. Van Poppel H, Da Pozzo L, Albrecht W, et al. A prospective, randomised EORTC intergroup phase 3 study comparing the oncologic outcome of elective nephron-sparing surgery and radical nephrectomy for low-stage renal cell carcinoma. *Eur Urol.* 2011;59(4):543–552.

13. Clark PE, Schover LR, Uzzo RG, Hafez KS, Rybicki LA, Novick AC. Quality of life and psychological adaptation after surgical treatment for localized renal cell carcinoma: impact of the amount of remaining renal tissue. *Urology.* 2001;57(2):252–256.

14. Ficarra V, Novella G, Sarti A, et al. Psycho-social well-being and general health status after surgical treatment for localized renal cell carcinoma. *Int Urol Nephrol.* 2002;34(4):441–446.

15. Shinohara N, Harabayashi T, Sato S, Hioka T, Tsuchiya K, Koyanagi T. Impact of nephron-sparing surgery on quality of life in patients with localized renal cell carcinoma. *Eur Urol.* 2001;39(1):114–119.

16. Parker PA, Swartz R, Fellman B, et al. Comprehensive assessment of quality of life and psychosocial adjustment in patients with renal tumors undergoing open, laparoscopic and nephron sparing surgery. *J Urol.* 2012;187(3):822–826.

17. Lau W, Blute ML, Weaver AL, Torres VE, Zincke H. Matched comparison of radical nephrectomy vs nephron-sparing surgery in patients with unilateral renal cell carcinoma and a normal contralateral kidney. *Mayo Clin Proc.* 2000 Dec;75(12):1236–1242.

18. Robson CJ, Churchill BM, Anderson W. The results of radical nephrectomy for renal cell carcinoma. *J Urol.* 1969;101(3):297–301.

19. Skinner DG, Vermillion CD, Colvin RB. The surgical management of renal cell carcinoma. *J Urol.* 1972;107(5):705–710.

20. Robson CJ, Churchill BM, Anderson W. The results of radical nephrectomy for renal cell carcinoma. *Trans Am Assoc Genitourin Surg.* 1968;60:122–129.

21. Freedland SJ, Dekernion JB. Role of lymphadenectomy for patients undergoing radical nephrectomy for renal cell carcinoma. *Rev Urol.* 2003;5(3):191–195.

22. Chapin BF, Delacroix SE Jr, Wood CG. The role of lymph node dissection in renal cell carcinoma. *Int J Clin Oncol.* 2011;16(3):186–194.

23. Hemal AK, Kumar A, Kumar R, Wadhwa P, Seth A, Gupta NP. Laparoscopic versus open radical nephrectomy for large renal tumors: a long-term prospective comparison. *J Urol.* 2007;177(3):862–866.

24. Permpongkosol S, Bagga HS, Romero FR, Sroka M, Jarrett TW, Kavoussi LR. Laparoscopic versus open partial nephrectomy for the treatment of pathological T1N0M0 renal cell carcinoma: a 5-year survival rate [see comment]. *J Urol.* 2006;176(5):1984–1988; discussion 1988–1989.

25. Hoang AN, Vaporcyian AA, Matin SF. Laparoscopy-assisted radical nephrectomy with inferior vena caval thrombectomy for level II to III tumor thrombus: a single-institution experience and review of the literature. *J Endourol.* 2010;24(6):1005–1012.

26. Matin SF, Abreu S, Ramani A, et al. Evaluation of age and comorbidity as risk factors after laparoscopic urological surgery. *J Urol.* 2003;170 (4 Pt 1):1115–1120.

27. Hsu TH, Gill IS, Fazeli-Matin S, et al. Radical nephrectomy and nephroureterectomy in the octogenarian and nonagenarian: comparison of laparoscopic and open approaches. *Urology.* 1999;53(6):1121–1125.

28. Matin SF, Madsen LT, Wood CG. Laparoscopic cytoreductive nephrectomy: the M. D. Anderson Cancer Center experience. *Urology.* 2006;68(3):528–532.

29. Walther MM, Lyne JC, Libutti SK, Linehan WM. Laparoscopic cytoreductive nephrectomy as preparation for administration of systemic interleukin-2 in the treatment of metastatic renal cell carcinoma: a pilot study. *Urology.* 1999;53(3):496–501.

30. Hollenbeck BK, Taub DA, Miller DC, Dunn RL, Wei JT. National utilization trends of partial nephrectomy for renal cell carcinoma: a case of underutilization? *Urology.* 2006;67(2):254–259.

31. Miller DC, Hollingsworth JM, Hafez KS, Daignault S, Hollenbeck BK. Partial nephrectomy for small renal masses: an emerging quality of care concern? *J Urol.* 2006;175(3 Pt 1):853–857; discussion 858.

32. Go AS, Chertow GM, Fan D, McCulloch CE, Hsu CY. Chronic kidney disease and the risks of death, cardiovascular events, and hospitalization. *N Engl J Med.* 2004;351(13):1296–1305.

33. Gill IS, Matin SF, Desai MM, et al. Comparative analysis of laparoscopic versus open partial nephrectomy for renal tumors in 200 patients. *J Urol.* 2003;170(1):64–68.

34. Benway BM, Bhayani SB, Rogers CG, et al. Robot assisted partial nephrectomy versus laparoscopic partial nephrectomy for renal tumors: a multi-institutional analysis of perioperative outcomes [see comment]. *J Urol.* 2009;182(3):866–872.

35. Faria E, Caputo P, Wood C, Karam J, Nogueras-Gonzalez G, Matin SF. Robotic partial nephrectomy shortens warm ischemia time, reducing suturing time kinetics even for an experienced laparoscopic surgeon: a comparative analysis. *World J Urol.* 2014;32(1):265–271.

Chapter 7

Staging and Surgical Management of Locally Advanced Renal Cell Carcinoma and the Role of Adjuvant and Neoadjuvant Therapy

Dae Y. Kim, Jose A. Karam, and Christopher G. Wood

Introduction

It is estimated that there will be 63,920 new cases of kidney and renal pelvis tumors with 13,860 deaths in the United States in 2014.[1] The lifetime risk of developing renal cell carcinoma (RCC) is 1 in 62, with major vein involvement (renal vein and inferior vena cava) occurring in 4%–10% of cases and metastatic spread in as many as 40%.[2] For patients who undergo surgery with curative intent, approximately 30% develop recurrence. Therefore, the management of patients with RCC involves a multidisciplinary approach with proper staging, risk stratification, surgery, and systemic therapy when indicated.

Staging

The most current staging system defines RCC tumor within the confines of the kidney as T1 and T2 disease and tumor extending beyond the kidney is ≥T3 (Table 7.1).[3] A T1a tumor is ≤4cm and a T1b tumor is between 4 and 7cm in diameter. Tumors larger than 7cm and smaller than 10cm are classified as T2a, and tumors measuring >10cm and confined to the kidney are classified as T2b. There are three sub-classifications of T3 disease, with T3a defined as tumor extending into the renal vein only or tumor extending into perinephric or sinus fat and limited within Gerota's fascia. The extension of thrombus into the inferior vena cava (IVC) and below the diaphragm is classified as T3b, with extension above the diaphragm or spread into the walls of

Table 7.1 2010 American Joint Committee on Cancer Staging System for Renal Cell Carcinoma

Primary Tumor (T)

TX Primary tumor cannot be assessed

T0 No evidence of primary tumor

T1 Tumor 7 cm or less in greatest dimension, limited to the kidney

T1a Tumor 4 cm or less in greatest dimension, limited to the kidney

T1b Tumor more than 4 cm but not more than 7 cm in greatest dimension limited to the kidney

T2 Tumor more than 7 cm in greatest dimension, limited to the kidney

T2a Tumor more than 7 cm but less than or equal to 10 cm in greatest dimension, limited to the kidney

T2b Tumor more than 10 cm, limited to the kidney

T3 Tumor extends into major veins or perinephric tissues but not into the ipsilateral adrenal gland and not beyond Gerota's fascia

T3a Tumor grossly extends into the renal vein or its segmental (muscle containing) branches, or tumor invades perirenal and/or renal sinus fat but not beyond Gerota's fascia

T3b Tumor grossly extends into the vena cava below the diaphragm

T3c Tumor grossly extends into the vena cava above the diaphragm or invades the wall of the vena cava

T4 Tumor invades beyond Gerota's fascia (including contiguous extension into the ipsilateral adrenal gland)

Regional Lymph Nodes (N)

NX Regional lymph nodes cannot be assessed

N0 No regional lymph node metastasis

N1 Metastasis in regional lymph node(s)

Distant Metastasis (M)

M0 No distant metastasis

M1 Distant metastasis

Anatomic Stage/Prognostic Groups

Stage I	T1	N0	M0
Stage II	T2	N0	M0
Stage III	T1 or T2	N1	M0
	T3	N0 or N1	M0
Stage IV	T4	Any N	M0
	Any T	Any N	M1

Source: Edge SB, American Joint Committee on Cancer. American Cancer Society. *AJCC Cancer Staging Handbook: from the AJCC Cancer Staging Manual.* 7th ed. New York: Springer; 2010.

the IVC defined as T3c disease. T4 disease describes tumor extending beyond Gerota's fascia or ipsilateral direct adrenal gland invasion.

Regional lymph nodes (LNs) are designated as N1 when they are involved, and distant metastasis is designated as M1. The tumor, nodal, and metastasis (TNM) staging system incorporates prognostic groups that describe stage I as T1, N0, and M0 and stage II as T2, N0, and M0. The 5-year cause-specific

Table 7.2 Venous Thrombus Staging Systems for Renal Cell Carcinoma

Landmark	Staging Systems				
	TNM (2010)[3]	Neves[5]	Novick[6]	Hinman[7]	Robson[8]
RV	T3a	0	I	I	
IVC <2cm above RV		I			
IVC >2cm above RV	T3b	II	II		IIIA
IVC at hepatic veins		III	III	II	
Above diaphragm	T3c	IV	IV	III	

Source: Adapted from Pouliot et al. *J Urol* 184 (3): 833–841, September 2010.[31]
IVC, inferior vena cava; RV, renal vein.

survival for stage I and II disease is 92.8%.[4] Stage III includes either T1 or T2 and N1 without distant metastasis (M0) or T3 with (N0) or without nodal (N1) involvement and without distant metastasis (M0). Stage IV describes T4 disease without distant metastasis or any T disease with distant metastasis (M1). The 5-year survival is 64.2% for stage III disease and 11.9% for stage IV disease.[4]

The extension of the venous thrombus (VT) is staged depending on its location (Table 7.2). Classification systems have been proposed by Neves,[5] Novick,[6] Hinman,[7] and Robson.[8] The VT at the height of the hepatic veins is classified as III, and above the diaphragm as IV using the Neves and Novick classifications. Stage II for Novick and Neves includes more than 2cm above the renal vein. Stage I for Neves includes less than 2cm above the renal vein, and stage 0 when the renal vein is included. For the Novick classification, stage I includes VT within the renal vein and up to 2 cm from the renal vein ostium. The Hinman classification includes stage I for extension into the IVC of more than 2cm, stage II for extension to the hepatic veins, and stage III for extension above the diaphragm. The Robson classification marks VT to the renal vein and IVC as stage IIIA, without distinction in the cephalad extent of tumor.

Imaging

To properly assess the stage of RCC, the extent of tumor burden, and distant metastasis, it is crucial to obtain the appropriate imaging studies prior to therapeutic intervention. The widespread availability of computed tomography (CT) has made it the initial diagnostic modality of choice. A VT should be suspected with the presence of lower extremity edema, varicocele, pulmonary embolism, dilated superficial veins, and a filling defect in the IVC or right atrium. Therefore, for locally advanced disease (T3 and higher), it is important to assess the extension of VT or invasion into the vena cava for proper staging and intervention.

The current imaging modality of choice for assessing extension of VT in the major vessels is magnetic resonance imaging (MRI). MR venography allows the accentuation of venous anatomy to assist in further surgical planning and interventions including venovenous bypass, cardiopulmonary bypass, and permissive hypothermic arrest. Recent advancements in multi-detector CT with reconstruction of images have increased the sensitivity of CT for detecting and correctly staging VT involvement.[9] Although MRI is currently the preferred method, patient-related restrictions such as metal implants, gadolinium allergy, and severe claustrophobia with prolonged scanning durations, may restrict its use and compel the use of CT.

If MRI and CT imaging are contraindicated or limited in their use and further characterization is desired, invasive venography may also be considered. Ultrasound is another modality used to characterize renal masses; however, its use preoperatively is limited in assessing VT extent. Transesophageal echocardiography is used intraoperatively to provide real-time assessment of VT in the right atrium, to monitor for dislodgement or retraction, and to confirm complete removal.

Prognostic Factors

Patient, surgical, and pathological characteristics are prognostic indicators that affect survival in RCC. Prognostic models that incorporate compromised performance/functional status, serum laboratory abnormalities ($\uparrow$lactate dehydrogenase, $\uparrow$Ca^{++}), higher T stage of tumor with presence of nodal and metastatic disease, presence of necrosis or sarcomatoid features, and fat invasion portend a worse prognosis.[10] Outcome prediction models have been developed for clear-cell renal cell carcinoma (ccRCC) after radical nephrectomy (RN) to estimate cancer-specific survival based on tumor stage, size, grade, and necrosis (SSIGN score).[11] The University of California–Los Angeles integrated staging system integrates the clinical variables of TNM stage, Fuhrman grade, and Eastern Cooperative Oncology Group performance status into five survival stratification groups.[12,13]

Surgical Management of Locally Advanced Renal Cell Carcinoma

Several approaches can be used to provide the necessary exposure for excising the mass including anterior, lateral, and posterior approaches as well as open, laparoscopic, and robotic approaches. Common surgical incisions for locally advanced RCC include midline, subcostal (or bilateral Chevron), thoracoabdominal, and flank approaches. A midline incision allows access to the kidneys as well as the major vessels and renal hilum. The subcostal and Chevron incisions provide adequate exposure for large tumors with bilateral renal hilar control. This incision is also optimal for hepatic mobilization for higher-level VT when the incision is extended into the midline to the thorax. The thoracoabdominal exposure is ideal for upper pole tumors and also provides accessibility to the renal hilum and retrohepatic IVC. If needed, the triangular and coronary ligaments of the liver (Langenbeck maneuver) are transected to provide hepatic mobility medially and cephalad for retrohepatic IVC exposure. The flank approach with either intercostal or transection of rib is used for tumors and VT limited to the renal vein and infrahepatic IVC.

Surgery for RCC with VT includes isolation and control of hilar vessels with early transection of the renal artery. The IVC is mobilized caudal and cephalad to the renal hilar vasculature with isolation of the contralateral renal vein. The venous structures are sequentially occluded cephalad to the VT, the contralateral renal vein, and the caudal IVC. A cavotomy is performed, along with excision of the renal vein ostium en-bloc with the specimen, and the VT is extracted completely followed by nephrectomy. The cavotomy is then closed or reconstructed either primarily or with patch grafts when the lumen is smaller than 50% of the original IVC diameter. In severe cases of VT invasion into the wall, en-bloc removal of the IVC dictates the use of biological or synthetic grafts.

For higher-level VT, venous bypass maneuvers have been implemented to maintain venous return to vital structures. For these maneuvers, a highly skilled team of anesthesiologists and urologic, vascular, hepatobiliary, and cardiothoracic surgeons is assembled. For cardiopulmonary bypass (CPB), the aortic arch or right subclavian artery, superior vena cava, and femoral vein are cannulized to provide the bypass circuit. Venovenous bypass is an alternative to CPB for lower-level tumors, primarily those that do not involve the right atrium. The venous system is cannulated distal and proximal to the VT in order to provide the bypass circuit, yielding shorter bypass, operative, and anesthesia times as compared with CPB.

Lymphadenectomy

Lymphadenectomy (LNTY) at the time of nephrectomy is the most reliable method for accurate staging and detection of LN metastasis. However, the therapeutic role of LN removal remains a matter of debate. The European Organization for Research and Treatment of Cancer, Genitourinary Group 30881, examined the role of LNTY for N0M0 disease randomized to RN with complete LNTY to RN alone.[14] A total of 772 patients were selected for randomization (383 LNTY + RN, 389 RN, 40 ineligible) with the majority of these patients (approximately 70%) having low clinical stage disease (≤T2). No differences in overall survival, time to progression, and progression-free survival were noted for the LNTY group. In total, only 4% of patients without clinically detectable LN demonstrated LN metastasis, and even with clinically detectable nodes, only 20% were positive for LN metastasis. For low clinical stage tumors without palpable LN (N0) and in the absence of high-risk features, LNTY may be of limited value.

Predicting LN involvement in locally advanced disease may dictate the therapeutic role of LNTY at the time of nephrectomy through complete resection of disease. The following five independent risk factors were identified that predict regional LN involvement: Fuhrman grade 3–4, sarcomatoid features, tumor size ≥10cm, tumor stage pT3-4, and presence of coagulative necrosis.[15] With zero or one risk factor, 6 of 1031 (0.6%) patients demonstrated LN metastasis, whereas with two risk factors, 62 of 621(10%) patients demonstrated spread to regional LN; when all five risk features were present, there was a 50% risk of regional LN involvement.

Neoadjuvant Therapy for Locally Advanced Renal Cell Carcinoma

Several case reports and case series have shown that the use of targeted therapies can convert locally advanced RCC from unresectable to resectable tumors (Table 7.3). Among 19 patients deemed to have unresectable disease, Thomas et al. demonstrated the feasibility of completing nephrectomy without surgical morbidity in 4 patients following neoadjuvant sunitinib therapy.[16] Amin et al. described nine patients with different RCC histological subtypes who achieved a mean decrease of 12.9% in size of the primary tumor, with operative outcomes similar to those of historical cohorts.[17] In another series with 30 patients (17 with localized disease), Cowey et al. examined the role of presurgical sorafenib with similar findings.[18]

Another potential advantage of neoadjuvant therapy for locally advanced RCC is reduction in tumor size, which facilitates nephron-sparing surgery (NSS). Hellenthal et al. treated 17 ccRCC patients with sunitinib and demonstrated a significant reduction in tumor size, facilitating NSS.[19] Shuch et al. described four patients whose primary tumor regressed after neoadjuvant targeted therapy to perform NSS.[20]

Adjuvant Therapy for Locally Advanced Renal Cell Carcinoma

To date, radiotherapy, hormonal therapy, immunotherapy, and chemotherapy is lacking in level 1 evidence to demonstrate benefit in the adjuvant setting (Table 7.3). Two studies (total 172 patients) examined the role of radiotherapy to the tumor bed after surgery for localized RCC and showed no differences in survival or relapse rates versus observation.[21,22] Tegafur-uracil, an oral 5-flourouracil prodrug, demonstrated no significant difference in the 5-year relapse-free rate versus observation.[23]

With the benefits of immunotherapy documented in metastatic RCC (mRCC), studies investigated the role of cytokines and vaccines to stimulate the host immune response after resection of locally advanced RCC. One study examined the role of interferon-alpha versus observation and showed similar 5-year overall survival (OS) rates (66.5% versus 66.0%).[24] In another study, a trend toward increased median OS was observed (5.1 years versus 7.4 years; $P = 0.09$).[25] In patients with resected locally advanced disease (T3b-4 or N1-3) or resected metastases (M1), one course of high-dose bolus interleukin-2 did not demonstrate significant survival benefit versus observation, with median disease-free survival of 28 months versus 20.5 months ($P = 0.7$), respectively.[26]

Table 7.3 Neoadjuvant and Adjuvant Studies in Locally Advanced Renal Cell Carcinoma

Reference	Trial Type	Therapy	Number of Patients	Measurement/Outcome	P Value
Neoadjuvant					
16	Retrospective	Sunitinib for 6-week cycle and for 4 consecutive weeks	19 patients; 4 underwent resection of tumor	Overall tumor partial response 2/19 (11%). 7/19 (37%) stable disease, 10/19 (53%) with disease progression; grade 3–4 toxicity in 37%	Not reported
17	Retrospective	Sunitinib (3 patients), sorafenib (5 patients), interferon + sorafenib (1 patient)	9 patients, unknown stage	Tumor shrinkage in all from 0.82% to 54%	Not reported
18	Prospective, nonrandomized	Sorafenib twice daily, median of 33-day administration	30 patients: 17 localized. 13 metastatic	23/30 with tumor shrinkage, 5/30 growth, 2/30 stable disease; no adverse surgical complications attributable to sorafenib	Not reported
19	Prospective, nonrandomized	Sunitinib for 90 days before nephrectomy	20 patients: 16 localized, 4 metastatic	17/20 (85%) with tumor shrinkage; grade 3 toxicity in 6 patients (30%); no adverse surgical	Not reported
Adjuvant					
21	RCT	Adjuvant radiotherapy to renal bed, incision, and para-aortic nodes vs observation	100	No significant difference in recurrence, metastases, or survival	NS

(Continued)

Table 7.3 (Continued)

Reference	Trial Type	Therapy	Number of Patients	Measurement/Outcome	P Value
22	RCT	Adjuvant radiation therapy to kidney bed vs observation	72	Median survival (50%) in adjuvant radiotherapy group = 26 months vs observation = 62% in 26 months	NS
23	RCT	Tegafur:uracil mixture vs observation	71	5-year nonrecurrence rate, 80.5% adjuvant vs 77.1 nonadjuvant	NS
24	RCT	IFN-α vs observation	247	5-year OS, 0.665 vs 0.660; event-free survival probabilities, 0.671 vs 0.567	NS
25	RCT	IFN-α vs observation	283	Median follow-up at 10.4 years median survival, 5.1 years vs 7.4 years	0.09
26	RCT	Single high-dose IL-2 vs observation	69	Median disease-free survival for high risk, locally advanced disease, 28 months vs 20.5 months	0.73
27	RCT	Intradermal injection of autologous irradiated tumor cells with bacille Calmette-Guérin vs observation	120	5-year OS, 69 vs 78; disease-free survival, 63 vs 72	NS

28	RCT	Autologous renal cell tumor vaccine vs observation	558 randomly allocated (379 eligible)	5-year progression-free survival, 67.5 vs 49.7	0.039
29	Retrospective	Autologous renal cell tumor vaccine vs observation	495 matched pairs	5-year OS, 71.3 vs 65.4; 10-year OS, 53.6 vs 36.2;	0.022
30	RCT	Tumor-derived heat shock protein complex (vitespan) vs observation	818	Recurrence events with median follow-up 1.9 years, 37.7 vs 39.8	0.506

IFN-α, interferon alpha; IL-2, interleukin-2; RCT, randomized controlled trial; OS, overall survival; RFS, recurrence free survival; NS not significant.

The application of tumor vaccines with the goal of invoking an immune response toward RCC cells has also been applied in the adjuvant setting. One study, which used bacille Calmette-Guérin, reported a 5-year disease-free survival (DFS) rate of 63% versus 72% (P = not significant).[27] Contemporary studies included intradermal injections of autologous tumor vaccine and demonstrated a 5-year progression-free survival (PFS) that favored vaccine therapy.[28] Despite a benefit in PFS, this trial was criticized because a large number of patients who were assigned to observation were lost to follow-up. A subsequent retrospective matched-pair analysis of 495 participants who were reported with a median follow-up of 131 months demonstrated 5-year and 10-year OS rates of 71.3 months and 53.6 months in the study group and 65.4 months and 36.2 months in the control group (P = 0.022), respectively, for patients with pT3 disease.[29] An autologous, tumor-derived heat-shock protein (glycoprotein 96)–peptide complex (vitespan) was administered in the adjuvant setting to patients with locally advanced RCC at high risk of recurrence. The primary endpoint in this open-label trial was recurrence-free survival, after a median follow-up of 1.9 years, the recurrence rates were similar (37.7% in the vitespan group versus 39.8% in the observation group; P = 0.506).[30]

Currently, targeted therapies are being investigated in the adjuvant setting for those who have locally advanced disease or are at high risk of relapse (Table 7.4). The Adjuvant Sorafenib or Sunitinib for Unfavorable Renal Carcinoma (ASSURE; NCT00326898) study randomized 1923 patients to receive sunitinib, sorafenib, or placebo for 1year after radical or partial nephrectomy. The Everolimus for Renal Cancer Ensuing Surgical Therapy (EVEREST; NCT01120249) trial is randomizing patients to receive everolimus or placebo for 1year. In a study to evaluate Pazopanib as an Adjuvant Treatment for Localized Renal Cell Carcinoma (PROTECT; NCT01235962), patients are randomized to receive pazopanib or placebo for 1year. Another phase 3 study, compares 1year versus 3year of sorafenib versus placebo with resected primary renal cell carcinoma at high or intermediate risk of relapse (SORCE trial; NCT00492258). The Sunitinib Treatment of Renal Adjuvant Cancer trial (S-TRAC trial; NCT00375674) compares DFS and safety of sunitinib versus placebo in the adjuvant treatment of patients at high risk of recurrent kidney cancer after surgery. The tyrosine kinase inhibitor, axitinib, is also being evaluated in the adjuvant setting in a randomized phase 3 trial versus placebo (ATLAS trial; NCT01599754).

Conclusion

Locally advanced RCC is amenable to aggressive curative resection. To successfully treat locally advanced RCC, appropriate staging dictates treatment and planning with multimodal therapies. Significant surgical and medical advances have led to improved patient outcomes. Future studies will refine the integration of these interventions.

Table 7.4 Ongoing Clinical Trials Evaluating Adjuvant Therapies for Locally Advanced and High-Risk Renal Cell Carcinoma

Trial	Study Design/Intervention	Inclusion Criteria	Endpoint	Primary Completion Date*
Sorafenib in treating patients at risk of relapse after undergoing surgery to remove kidney cancer (SORCE; NCT00492258)	RCT: 1656 patients Treatment arm 1: Placebo arm 2: sorafenib for 1 year, placebo for 2 years Arm 3: sorafenib for 3 years, if progression in arm 1 and arm 2 crossover to arm 3	ccRCC and non-ccRCC; intermediate or high risk; surgery for RCC; no residual disease	Primary: DFS Secondary: metastasis-free survival, OS, cost-effectiveness, toxicity	August 2012
Sunitinib vs placebo for the treatment of patients at high risk of recurrent renal cell cancer (Sunitinib Treatment of Renal Adjuvant Cancer trial; S-TRAC; NCT00375674)	RCT: 720 patients Treatment: sunitinib vs placebo	Predominant ccRCC; high risk renal cancer; ECOG-PS 0–2; kidney tumor removed; no macroscopic disease	Primary: DFS Secondary: OS, safety, tolerability, patient-reported outcomes	November 2015
Sunitinib or Sorafenib in treating patients with kidney cancer that was removed by surgery (The Adjuvant Sorafenib or Sunitinib for Unfavorable Renal carcinoma; ASSURE NCT00326898)	RCT: 1923 patients Treatment with sunitinib, sorafenib, and placebo; treatment to start 4–12 weeks after radical and partial nephrectomy	ccRCC and non-ccRCC; intermediate or high risk (pT1b-pT3a, N0, M0); very high risk (pT3a-pT4, N0, M0, pT any, N+, M0)	Primary: DFS Secondary: OS, DFS with ccRCC, cardiac parameters, quality of life	April 2016
A study to evaluate pazopanib as an adjuvant treatment for localized RCC (PROTECT; NCT01235962)	RCT:1500 patients Arm 1: pazopanib Arm 2: placebo	ccRCC or predominant ccRCC; pT2 (G3-4)–pT4 (any G, N0) or pT (any G any, N1, all M0)	Primary: DFS Secondary: OS, safety, and health outcomes	October 2016

(Continued)

Table 7.4 (Continued)

Trial	Study Design/Intervention	Inclusion Criteria	Endpoint	Primary Completion Date*
Adjuvant axitinib therapy for RCC in high-risk patients (ATLAS; NCT01599754)	RCT: 592 patients Treatment: axitinib vs placebo	Predominant ccRCC; no macroscopic or metastatic disease; pT2–T4 (pT3a > 4cm), Nx, M0; ECOG-PS 0–1	Primary: DFS Secondary: OS, safety	June 2017
Everolimus in treating patients with kidney cancer who have undergone surgery (Everolimus for Renal Cancer Ensuing Surgical Therapy; EVEREST; NCT01120249)	RCT: 1218 patients Arm 1: everolimus Arm 2: placebo	ccRCC and non-ccRCC; intermediate high risk or very high risk; have undergone full resection and without metastatic disease	Primary: RFS Secondary: OS and toxicity	October 2021

ccRCC, clear-cell renal cell carcinoma; DFS, disease-free survival; ECOG-PS, Eastern Cooperative Oncology Group–Performance Status; OS, overall survival; RCC, renal cell carcinoma; RCT, randomized controlled trial.

* Final data collection date for primary outcome measure.

References

1. Siegel R, Ma J, Zou Z, Jemal A. Cancer statistics, 2014. *CA: A Cancer Journal for Clinicians.* Jan–Feb 2014;64(1):9–29.

2. Kenney PA, Wood CG. Integration of surgery and systemic therapy for renal cell carcinoma. *The Urologic Clinics of North America.* May 2012;39(2):211–231, vii.

3. Edge SB, American Joint Committee on Cancer., American Cancer Society. *AJCC cancer staging handbook : from the AJCC cancer staging manual.* 7th ed. New York: Springer; 2010.

4. Sun M, Thuret R, Abdollah F, et al. Age-adjusted incidence, mortality, and survival rates of stage-specific renal cell carcinoma in North America: a trend analysis. *European urology.* Jan 2011;59(1):135–141.

5. Neves RJ, Zincke H. Surgical treatment of renal cancer with vena cava extension. *British journal of urology.* May 1987;59(5):390–395.

6. Glazer A, Novick AC. Preoperative transesophageal echocardiography for assessment of vena caval tumor thrombi: a comparative study with venacavography and magnetic resonance imaging. *Urology.* Jan 1997;49(1):32–34.

7. Hinman F. *Atlas of urologic surgery.* 2nd ed. Philadelphia: W.B. Saunders; 1998.

8. Robson CJ, Churchill BM, Anderson W. The results of radical nephrectomy for renal cell carcinoma. *The Journal of urology.* Mar 1969;101(3):297–301.

9. Lawrentschuk N, Gani J, Riordan R, Esler S, Bolton DM. Multidetector computed tomography vs magnetic resonance imaging for defining the upper limit of tumour thrombus in renal cell carcinoma: a study and review. *BJU international.* Aug 2005;96(3):291–295.

10. Sorbellini M, Kattan MW, Snyder ME, et al. A postoperative prognostic nomogram predicting recurrence for patients with conventional clear cell renal cell carcinoma. *The Journal of urology.* Jan 2005;173(1):48–51.

11. Frank I, Blute ML, Cheville JC, Lohse CM, Weaver AL, Zincke H. An outcome prediction model for patients with clear cell renal cell carcinoma treated with radical nephrectomy based on tumor stage, size, grade and necrosis: the SSIGN score. *The Journal of urology.* Dec 2002;168(6):2395–2400.

12. Patard JJ, Kim HL, Lam JS, et al. Use of the University of California Los Angeles integrated staging system to predict survival in renal cell carcinoma: an international multicenter study. *Journal of clinical oncology : official journal of the American Society of Clinical Oncology.* Aug 15 2004;22(16):3316–3322.

13. Zisman A, Pantuck AJ, Dorey F, et al. Improved prognostication of renal cell carcinoma using an integrated staging system. *Journal of clinical oncology : official journal of the American Society of Clinical Oncology.* Mar 15 2001;19(6):1649–1657.

14. Blom JH, van Poppel H, Marechal JM, et al. Radical nephrectomy with and without lymph-node dissection: final results of European Organization for Research and Treatment of Cancer (EORTC) randomized phase 3 trial 30881. *European urology.* Jan 2009;55(1):28–34.

15. Blute ML, Leibovich BC, Cheville JC, Lohse CM, Zincke H. A protocol for performing extended lymph node dissection using primary tumor pathological features for patients treated with radical nephrectomy for clear cell renal cell carcinoma. *The Journal of urology.* Aug 2004;172(2):465–469.

16. Thomas AA, Rini BI, Lane BR, et al. Response of the primary tumor to neoadjuvant sunitinib in patients with advanced renal cell carcinoma. *The Journal of urology.* Feb 2009;181(2):518–523; discussion 523.

17. Amin C, Wallen E, Pruthi RS, Calvo BF, Godley PA, Rathmell WK. Preoperative tyrosine kinase inhibition as an adjunct to debulking nephrectomy. *Urology.* Oct 2008;72(4):864–868.

18. Cowey CL, Amin C, Pruthi RS, et al. Neoadjuvant clinical trial with sorafenib for patients with stage II or higher renal cell carcinoma. *Journal of clinical oncology : official journal of the American Society of Clinical Oncology.* Mar 20 2010;28(9):1502–1507.

19. Hellenthal NJ, Underwood W, Penetrante R, et al. Prospective clinical trial of preoperative sunitinib in patients with renal cell carcinoma. *The Journal of urology.* Sep 2010;184(3):859–864.

20. Shuch B, Riggs SB, LaRochelle JC, et al. Neoadjuvant targeted therapy and advanced kidney cancer: observations and implications for a new treatment paradigm. *BJU international.* Sep 2008;102(6):692–696.

21. Finney R. The value of radiotherapy in the treatment of hypernephroma--a clinical trial. *British journal of urology.* Jun 1973;45(3):258–269.

22. Kjaer M, Frederiksen PL, Engelholm SA. Postoperative radiotherapy in stage II and III renal adenocarcinoma. A randomized trial by the Copenhagen Renal Cancer Study Group. *International journal of radiation oncology, biology, physics.* May 1987;13(5):665–672.

23. Naito S, Kumazawa J, Omoto T, et al. Postoperative UFT adjuvant and the risk factors for recurrence in renal cell carcinoma: a long-term follow-up study. Kyushu University Urological Oncology Group. *International journal of urology: official journal of the Japanese Urological Association.* Jan 1997;4(1):8–12.

24. Pizzocaro G, Piva L, Colavita M, et al. Interferon adjuvant to radical nephrectomy in Robson stages II and III renal cell carcinoma: a multicentric randomized study. *Journal of clinical oncology : official journal of the American Society of Clinical Oncology.* Jan 15 2001;19(2):425–431.

25. Messing EM, Manola J, Wilding G, et al. Phase III study of interferon alfa-NL as adjuvant treatment for resectable renal cell carcinoma: an Eastern Cooperative Oncology Group/Intergroup trial. *Journal of clinical oncology : official journal of the American Society of Clinical Oncology.* Apr 1 2003;21(7):1214–1222.

26. Clark JI, Atkins MB, Urba WJ, et al. Adjuvant high-dose bolus interleukin-2 for patients with high-risk renal cell carcinoma: a cytokine working group randomized trial. *Journal of clinical oncology : official journal of the American Society of Clinical Oncology.* Aug 15 2003;21(16):3133–3140.

27. Galligioni E, Quaia M, Merlo A, et al. Adjuvant immunotherapy treatment of renal carcinoma patients with autologous tumor cells and bacillus Calmette-Guerin: five-year results of a prospective randomized study. *Cancer.* Jun 15 1996;77(12):2560–2566.

28. Jocham D, Richter A, Hoffmann L, et al. Adjuvant autologous renal tumour cell vaccine and risk of tumour progression in patients with renal-cell carcinoma after radical nephrectomy: phase III, randomised controlled trial. *Lancet.* Feb 21 2004;363(9409):594–599.

29. May M, Brookman-May S, Hoschke B, et al. Ten-year survival analysis for renal carcinoma patients treated with an autologous tumour lysate vaccine in an adjuvant setting. *Cancer immunology, immunotherapy : CII.* May 2010;59(5):687–695.

30. Wood C, Srivastava P, Bukowski R, et al. An adjuvant autologous therapeutic vaccine (HSPPC-96; vitespen) versus observation alone for patients at high

risk of recurrence after nephrectomy for renal cell carcinoma: a multicentre, open-label, randomised phase III trial. *Lancet*. Jul 12 2008;372(9633):145–154.

31. Pouliot F, Shuch B, Larochelle JC, Pantuck A, Belldegrun AS. Contemporary management of renal tumors with venous tumor thrombus. *The Journal of urology*. Sep 2010;184(3):833–841; quiz 1235.

Chapter 8

Integration of Targeted Therapy with Cytoreductive Nephrectomy and Metastasectomy in the Management of Metastatic Renal Cell Carcinoma

Bishoy A. Gayed, Jose A. Karam, Vitaly Margulis, and Christopher G. Wood

Introduction

Surgical resection is currently the mainstay treatment for localized renal cell carcinoma (RCC). However, for patients with metastatic RCC (mRCC), surgery alone has limited benefits and may only be curative if all metastatic deposits are excised.[1,2] The combination of surgery and systemic therapy for the treatment of advanced RCC is required to halt disease progression and improve overall survival.

In recent years, a shift in the management paradigm of advanced RCC has occurred as a result of an improved understanding of RCC tumor biology. Development of receptor tyrosine kinase inhibitors (TKIs), vascular endothelial growth factor (VEGF) antibodies, and mammalian target of rapamycin (mTORs) inhibitors have translated into significant benefits over cytokine therapy and have become mainstays of systemic treatments for mRCC.[3]

While cytoreductive nephrectomy (CN) has shown benefit in improving oncologic outcomes in patients with mRCC, its timing in the era of targeted agents remains undefined. Several studies have shown improvements in oncological outcomes for the presurgical use of targeted agents followed by CN and for upfront CN followed by targeted agents.[4–6] Herein, we discuss the rationale, patient selection, and outcomes of these approaches. Further, we discuss the role of metastasectomy in the era of targeted agents.

Cytoreductive Nephrectomy

Evidence for the role of CN stems from two randomized phase 3 clinical trials conducted in patients with mRCC in the cytokine era. Southwest Oncology Group (SWOG) 8949 randomized 241 patients to either CN followed by interferon alpha-2b (INFα-2b) or INFα alone.[7] Results showed a significant improvement in overall survival (OS) in patients undergoing CN versus INFα alone (11.1 months versus 8.1 months). Additionally, long-term results of the study continued to show that patients randomized to nephrectomy had improved OS.[8]

The European Organization for Research and Treatment of Cancer (EORTC-30947) randomized 85 patients with mRCC to receive CN + INFα versus INFα alone.[9] Again, a significant benefit was seen in OS in the CN + INFα group versus the INFα group (17 months versus 7 months).[9] In a pooled analysis of both trials, the CN + INFα group continued to show improvement in OS (13.6 months versus 7.8 months).[10]

There are several theories that explain the benefit of CN in patients with mRCC. These theories focus mainly on the immune dysfunctions associated with RCC.[11] Primary tumors are theorized to act as an "immunologic sink," depleting antibodies and lymphocytes.[11,12]

Additionally, the primary tumor is thought to secrete proangiogenic factors such as VEGF and basic fibroblast growth factor (bFGF), which contribute to progression and metastatic deposits.[13] Thus, removal of the primary tumor, in theory, may remove these factors and limit the spread of metastasis. While several theories explain the biological benefit of CN, this benefit most likely is a result of a decrease in tumor burden coupled with restoration of angiogenic balance.[14]

With an immunological and a clinical benefit of CN being apparent in patients receiving cytokine therapy, one can extrapolate that the same benefits would apply to the use of CN and targeted agents. Additionally, support for the use of targeted agents stems from trials that exposed patients to upfront CN followed by systemic therapy, thus possibly establishing CN as a prognostic factor.[15,16]

However, results from a recent SEER study revealed that the use of CN has actually declined since the introduction of targeted agents into clinical practice.[17] This could be due to several factors such as the uncertainty of CN in this era and concerns of delaying effective systemic therapy.

Patient Selection

Despite improvements in morbidity and mortality, CN can be technically difficult and is associated with nearly a 31% complication rate.[18] Additionally, a subset of patients will rapidly progress following nephrectomy and become ineligible for systemic therapy.[11] Stratification tools to determine which patients will benefit from CN versus those that will not benefit are lacking.

Multiple investigators have reported on several prognostic factors that have been identified to determine who will benefit from CN. Culp et al. retrospectively reviewed the records of 566 patients with mRCC.[19] On multivariate analysis, independent predictors of inferior OS included elevated serum lactate dehydrogenase level, decreased serum albumin level, symptomatic presentations by metastatic site, liver metastasis, retroperitoneal and supradiaphragmatic adenopathy, and clinical tumor classification >T3.[19] Surgical patients who had more than four risk factors did not appear to benefit from CN (Box 8.1).

Recently, Margulis et al. developed a predictive model to help guide selection of patients who would benefit from CN.[20] Using a cohort of 601 patients, several predictive factors were incorporated into a model to determine significance. Using variables such as serum albumin and serum lactate dehydrogenase levels and stage and node status, both preoperative and postoperative models were accurate predictors of cancer-specific survival (CSS) after CN.[20] However, these models still lack validation in independent series and thus their use is not widespread.

While we lack the tools to determine which patients will likely benefit from CN, several risk stratification models exist to predict survival in patients with mRCC.[14] Currently, the Memorial Sloan-Kettering Cancer Center (MSKCC) prognostic model is the most widely used risk model and was developed based on data from the cytokine era.[21] The MSKCC model incorporates factors that are independent predictors of poor outcome: low Karnofsky performance status, low hemoglobin, high lactate dehydrogenase, high corrected serum calcium, and lack of prior nephrectomy.[14] Based on the number of risk factors present, patients are stratified into three risk groups: good, intermediate, and poor, with median survival of 20 months, 10 months, and 4 months, respectively.[21,22]

Heng et al. validated the MSKCC model to predict OS in patients with mRCC treated with anti-VEGF agents and identified neutrophilia and thrombocytosis as additional risk factors.[23]

Box 8.1 Adverse Prognostic Factors for Inferior Overall Survival

- Low hemoglobin level
- Elevated lactate dehydrogenase
- Low albumin level
- Elevated corrected serum calcium level
- Symptoms due to metastases
- Liver, lung, retroperitoneal nodal metastases
- Clinical stage >T3
- Low Karnofsky performance status
- Absence of prior nephrectomy
- Time elapsed from diagnosis until treatment

Adapted from Abel and Wood 2009; Culp et al. 2010; Margulis et al. 2012; and Motzer et al. 2008.

Timing of Surgery

While the benefit of CN and targeted therapy has been shown in numerous studies, the optimal timing of CN has yet to be determined in the targeted therapy era.

Presurgical Targeted Therapy Followed by Cytoreductive Nephrectomy

In the era of targeted therapy, several studies have shown that patients may derive benefit from presurgical therapy with targeted agents followed by CN. In a recent retrospective study, Stroup et al. compared two groups of patients who underwent upfront CN followed by sunitinib (group 1) versus presurgical sunitinib followed by CN (group 2) and demonstrated significant improvement of disease-specific survival (DSS) and OS in favor of patients who underwent presurgical sunitinib therapy followed by CN. Further, 11/18 (61%) patients in group 2 had a partial response or stable disease in response to sunitinib.[24]

Wood and Margulis compared patients who received presurgical targeted therapy followed by CN versus patients who underwent upfront CN.[25] Both cohorts were matched in terms of clinical characteristics, tumor burden, and number of adverse prognostic factors. No significant difference between the two groups was found (27.7 months versus 31 months; $P = 0.697$).[25]

To better address the role of CN and its timing, EORTC 30073, the SURTIME trial, is currently enrolling patients with mRCC and primary tumor in situ to compare upfront CN followed by sunitinib versus sunitinib followed by CN.[26]

The rationale for the use of presurgical treatment stems from several potential benefits. One theoretical benefit is the ability to downsize tumors to facilitate surgery. Several groups have reported on the effect of targeted agents on the reduction of tumor size and the ability to convert tumors from unresectable to resectable disease (Table 8.1).[6,27–33]

Another potential benefit of presurgical therapy is expeditious initiation of systemic therapy. Further, presurgical therapy can serve as a "litmus test" for selecting patients who respond to therapy and are most likely to benefit from CN.[34]

However, presurgical therapy does have limitations. Presurgical therapy requires an accurate tissue diagnosis to determine histology. In a recent series of 405 preoperative biopsies in patients with mRCC, biopsy and nephrectomy specimens were correlated in only 72.7% of patients with non–clear-cell RCC and 96% with clear-cell RCC. Further, only 7/76 (9.2%) of the biopsies accurately identified sarcomatoid dedifferentiation.[35]

Further, presurgical therapy is associated with a delay in CN and may lead to disease progression. In addition, presurgical therapy has been associated with impaired tissue healing and preoperative bleeding and/or thromboembolic

Table 8.1 Studies Evaluating the Role of Presurgical Targeted Therapy and Effect on Tumor Size

Author	Study Type	Number of Patients	Therapy	Median Rate of Tumor Reduction, %
Thomas et al.[27]	Retrospective	19	Sunitinib	24
van der Veldt et al.[29]	Retrospective	22	Sunitinib	31
Abel et al.[35]	Retrospective	168	Multiple tyrosine kinase inhibitors	7.1
Jonasch et al.[30]	Prospective	50	Bevacizumab	12
Powles et al.[6]	Retrospective	52	Sunitinib	12
Silberstein et al.[31]	Retrospective	12	Sunitinib	21.1
Rini et al.[32]	Prospective	30	Sunitinib	22
Hellenthal et al.[28]	Prospective	20	Sunitinib	11.8
Cowey et al.[33]	Prospective	30	Sorafenib	9.6

phenomena.[36,37] However, several studies have shown that presurgical therapy is safe and does not increase surgical morbidity or perioperative complications when compared with upfront CN.[38,39]

Cytoreductive Nephrectomy Followed by Targeted Therapy

The current standard of CN followed by systemic therapy reflects the experience derived from the cytokine era. While targeted agents have become the mainstay of systemic therapy, the role of upfront CN has yet to be established.

Choueiri et al. evaluated 314 patients to determine the impact of CN on survival of patients with mRCC;[5] 201 patients underwent upfront CN and targeted therapy versus 113 patients who received targeted therapy alone. Median OS for those who underwent CN + targeted therapy was 19.8 months compared with 9.4 months for those who did not ($P < 0.01$). However, patients who had poor-risk disease received a marginal benefit from CN.[5,22]

In a retrospective study, You et al. evaluated 78 patients with mRCC to compare the effectiveness of CN and targeted agents; 45 patients underwent CN and received sunitinib or sorafenib and 33 patients received sunitinib or sorafenib without CN.[40] The median progression-free survival for the CN group was 11.7 months compared with 9.0 months for patients who received systemic therapy alone, with median OS of 21.6 months and 13.9 months, respectively. However, these differences did not reach statistical significance.[40]

Currently, the CARMENA trial (NCT00930033), a randomized phase 3 noninferiority trial, is comparing OS in patients treated with sunitinib alone versus CN followed by sunitinib.[22,41]

Metastasectomy

Historical evidence for the benefits of metastasectomy is derived from several retrospective series. Van der Poel et al. evaluated 152 resections of RCC metastases in 101 patients.[42] Median survival after metastasectomy was 28 months, and patients with a tumor-free interval of more than 2 years between initial nephrectomy and metastasis had a longer DSS.[42] Pogrebniak et al. evaluated the role of metastasectomy in survival of patients with isolated pulmonary metastases. Patients who underwent complete resection of their lesions had a longer survival compared with patients with incomplete resection of their lesions (49 months versus 16 months; $P = 0.02$). Their data support surgical resection of isolated metastatic disease from RCC.[43]

Recently, Eggener et al. retrospectively reviewed 129 patients with mRCC and showed that patients with oligometastatic disease who underwent metastasectomy appear to have a greater survival benefit.[44] Others have also described the impact of complete metastasectomy on improved CSS (4.8 years versus 1.3 years), even with multiple metastatic deposits.[45] However, at present, metastasectomy is reserved for patients with solitary or limited metastases when complete resection is feasible and for patients with metastases who demonstrate a response to systemic therapy.[46]

However, the role and timing of metastasectomy in patients receiving targeted therapies remains undefined. Yuasa et al. evaluated 139 metastatic sites and 16 primary lesions treated with sunitinib or sorafenib.[47] While the overall median tumor reduction rate was 23.8%, there was a significant reduction in the size of metastatic lesions compared with the primary tumor (43.2% versus 16.1%; $P < 0.001$).[47]

Recently, Karam et al. reported results of a retrospective study in patients undergoing metastasectomy after targeted therapy. Among 22 patients, 4 achieved a partial response, 11 had stable disease, and 4 progressed. At the time of analysis, 50% had recurred, while only one patient had died.[48] While this study showed that targeted therapy prior to metastasectomy is feasible and associated with low surgical morbidity, several questions about the role of targeted agents remain, including selection of the targeted agent and its treatment duration and whether or not to resume therapy postoperatively with the same agent or a new one.[48]

References

1. Gupta K, Miller JD, Li JZ, et al. Epidemiologic and socioeconomic burden of metastatic renal cell carcinoma (mRCC): a literature review. *Cancer Treat Rev.* 2008;34(3):193–205.

2. Ljungberg B, Hanbury DC, Kuczyk MA, et al. Renal cell carcinoma guideline. *Eur Urol.* 2007;51(6):1502–1510.

3. Patard JJ, Pignot G, Escudier B, et al. ICUD-EAU International Consultation on Kidney Cancer 2010: treatment of metastatic disease. *Eur Urol.* 2011;60(4):684–690.

4. Richey SL, Culp SH, Jonasch E, et al. Outcome of patients with metastatic renal cell carcinoma treated with targeted therapy without cytoreductive nephrectomy. *Ann Oncol.* 2011;22(5):1048–1053.

5. Choueiri TK, Xie W, Kollmannsberger C, et al. The impact of cytoreductive nephrectomy on survival of patients with metastatic renal cell carcinoma receiving vascular endothelial growth factor targeted therapy. *J Urol.* 2011;185(1):60–66.

6. Powles T, Blank C, Chowdhury S, et al. The outcome of patients treated with sunitinib prior to planned nephrectomy in metastatic clear cell renal cancer. *Eur Urol.* 2011;60(3):448–454.

7. Flanigan RC, Salmon SE, Blumenstein BA, et al. Nephrectomy followed by interferon alfa-2b compared with interferon alfa-2b alone for metastatic renal-cell cancer. *N Engl J Med.* 2001;6;345(23):1655–1659.

8. Lara PN, Jr., Tangen CM, Conlon SJ, et al. Predictors of survival of advanced renal cell carcinoma: long-term results from Southwest Oncology Group Trial S8949. *J Urol.* 2009;181(2):512–516; discussion 6–7.

9. Mickisch GH, Garin A, van Poppel H, et al. Radical nephrectomy plus interferon-alfa-based immunotherapy compared with interferon alfa alone in metastatic renal-cell carcinoma: a randomised trial. *Lancet.* 2001;22;358(9286):966–970.

10. Flanigan RC, Mickisch G, Sylvester R, et al. Cytoreductive nephrectomy in patients with metastatic renal cancer: a combined analysis. *J Urol.* 2004;171(3):1071–1076.

11. Abel EJ, Wood CG. Cytoreductive nephrectomy for metastatic RCC in the era of targeted therapy. *Nat Rev Urol.* 2009;6(7):375–383.

12. Robertson CN, Linehan WM, Pass HI, et al. Preparative cytoreductive surgery in patients with metastatic renal cell carcinoma treated with adoptive immunotherapy with interleukin-2 or interleukin-2 plus lymphokine activated killer cells. *J Urol.* 1990;144(3):614–617; discussion 7–8.

13. Slaton JW, Inoue K, Perrotte P, et al. Expression levels of genes that regulate metastasis and angiogenesis correlate with advanced pathological stage of renal cell carcinoma. *Am J Pathol.* 2001;158(2):735–743.

14. Margulis V, Wood CG, Jonasch E, et al. Current status of debulking nephrectomy in the era of tyrosine kinase inhibitors. *Curr Oncol Rep.* 2008;10(3):253–258.

15. Escudier B, Eisen T, Stadler WM, et al. Sorafenib for treatment of renal cell carcinoma: Final efficacy and safety results of the phase III treatment approaches in renal cancer global evaluation trial. *J Clin Oncol.* 2009;;27(20):3312–3318.

16. Motzer RJ, Hutson TE, Tomczak P, et al. Sunitinib versus interferon alfa in metastatic renal-cell carcinoma. *N Engl J Med.* 2007;356(2):115–124.

17. Tsao CK, Small AC, Kates M, et al. Cytoreductive nephrectomy for metastatic renal cell carcinoma in the era of targeted therapy in the United States: a SEER analysis. *World J Urol.* 2013;31(6):1535–1539.

18. Trinh QD, Bianchi M, Hansen J, et al. In-hospital mortality and failure to rescue after cytoreductive nephrectomy. *Eur Urol.* 2013;63(6):1107–1114.

19. Culp SH, Tannir NM, Abel EJ, et al. Can we better select patients with metastatic renal cell carcinoma for cytoreductive nephrectomy? *Cancer.* 2010;116 (14):3378–3388.

20. Margulis V, Shariat SF, Rapoport Y, et al. Development of accurate models for individualized prediction of survival after cytoreductive nephrectomy for metastatic renal cell carcinoma. *Eur Urol.* 2013;63(5):947–952.

21. Motzer RJ, Mazumdar M, Bacik J, et al. Survival and prognostic stratification of 670 patients with advanced renal cell carcinoma. *J Clin Oncol.* 1999;17(8):2530–2540.

22. Karam JA, Wood CG. The role of surgery in advanced renal cell carcinoma: cytoreductive nephrectomy and metastasectomy. *Hematol Oncol Clin North Am.* 2011;25(4):753–764.

23. Heng DY, Xie W, Regan MM, et al. Prognostic factors for overall survival in patients with metastatic renal cell carcinoma treated with vascular endothelial growth factor-targeted agents: results from a large, multicenter study. *J Clin Oncol.* 2009;27(34):5794–5799.

24. Stroup SP, Raheem OA, Palazzi KL, et al. Does timing of cytoreductive nephrectomy impact patient survival with metastatic renal cell carcinoma in the tyrosine kinase inhibitor era? A multi-institutional study. *Urology.* 2013;81(4):805–811.

25. Wood CG, Margulis V. Neoadjuvant (presurgical) therapy for renal cell carcinoma: a new treatment paradigm for locally advanced and metastatic disease. *Cancer.* 2009;115(10 Suppl):2355–2360.

26. Immediate surgery or surgery after sunitinib malate in treating patients with metastatic kidney cancer. US National Institutes of Health Web site: http://clinicaltrialsgov/ct2/show/NCT01099423.

27. Thomas AA, Rini BI, Lane BR, et al. Response of the primary tumor to neoadjuvant sunitinib in patients with advanced renal cell carcinoma. *J Urol.* 2009;181(2):518–523; discussion 23.

28. Hellenthal NJ, Underwood W, Penetrante R, et al. Prospective clinical trial of preoperative sunitinib in patients with renal cell carcinoma. *J Urol.* 2010;184(3):859–864.

29. van der Veldt AA, Meijerink MR, van den Eertwegh AJ, et al. Sunitinib for treatment of advanced renal cell carcinoma: primary tumor response. *Clin Cancer Res.* 2008;14(8):2431–2436.

30. Jonasch E, Wood CG, Matin SF, et al. Phase II presurgical feasibility study of bevacizumab in untreated patients with metastatic renal cell carcinoma. *J Clin Oncol.* 2009;27(25):4076–4081.

31. Silberstein JL, Millard F, Mehrazin R, et al. Feasibility and efficacy of neoadjuvant sunitinib before nephron-sparing surgery. *BJU Int.* 2010;106(9):1270–1276.

32. Rini BI, Garcia J, Elson P, et al. The effect of sunitinib on primary renal cell carcinoma and facilitation of subsequent surgery. *J Urol.* 2012;187(5):1548–1554.

33. Cowey CL, Amin C, Pruthi RS, et al. Neoadjuvant clinical trial with sorafenib for patients with stage II or higher renal cell carcinoma. *J clin ONcol.* 2010;28(9):1502–1507.

34. Margulis V, Wood CG. Cytoreductive nephrectomy in the era of targeted molecular agents: is it time to consider presurgical systemic therapy? *Eur Urol.* 2008;54(3):489–492.

35. Abel EJ, Carrasco A, Culp SH, et al. Limitations of preoperative biopsy in patients with metastatic renal cell carcinoma: comparison to surgical pathology in 405 cases. *BJU Int.* 2012;110(11):1742–1746.

36. Roman CD, Choy H, Nanney L, et al. Vascular endothelial growth factor-mediated angiogenesis inhibition and postoperative wound healing in rats. *J Surg Res.* 2002;105(1):43–47.

37. Margulis V, Wood CG. Pre-surgical targeted molecular therapy in renal cell carcinoma. *BJU Int.* 2009;103(2):150–153.

38. Margulis V, Matin SF, Tannir N, et al. Surgical morbidity associated with administration of targeted molecular therapies before cytoreductive nephrectomy or resection of locally recurrent renal cell carcinoma. *J Urol.* 2008;180(1):94–98.

39. Chapin BF, Delacroix SE, Jr., Culp SH, et al. Safety of presurgical targeted therapy in the setting of metastatic renal cell carcinoma. *Eur Urol.* 2011;60(5):964–971.

40. You D, Jeong IG, Ahn JH, et al. The value of cytoreductive nephrectomy for metastatic renal cell carcinoma in the era of targeted therapy. *J Urol.* 2011;185(1):54–59.

41. Bellmunt J. Future developments in renal cell carcinoma. *Ann Oncol.* 2009;20 Suppl 1:i13–i17.

42. van der Poel HG, Roukema JA, Horenblas S, et al. Metastasectomy in renal cell carcinoma: A multicenter retrospective analysis. *Eur Urol.* 1999;35(3):197–203.

43. Pogrebniak HW, Haas G, Linehan WM, et al. Renal cell carcinoma: resection of solitary and multiple metastases. *Ann Thorac Surg.* 1992;54(1):33–38.

44. Eggener SE, Yossepowitch O, Kundu S, et al. Risk score and metastasectomy independently impact prognosis of patients with recurrent renal cell carcinoma. *J Urol.* 2008;180(3):873–878; discussion 8.

45. Alt AL, Boorjian SA, Lohse CM, et al. Survival after complete surgical resection of multiple metastases from renal cell carcinoma. *Cancer.* 2011;117 (13):2873–2882.

46. Ljungberg B. The role of metastasectomy in renal cell carcinoma in the era of targeted therapy. *Curr Urol Rep.* 2013;14(1):19–25.

47. Yuasa T, Urakami S, Yamamoto S, et al. Tumor size is a potential predictor of response to tyrosine kinase inhibitors in renal cell cancer. *Urology.* 2011;77(4):831–835.

48. Karam JA, Rini BI, Varella L, et al. Metastasectomy after targeted therapy in patients with advanced renal cell carcinoma. *J Urol.* 2011;185(2):439–444.

Chapter 9

Immunotherapeutic Approaches for Metastatic Conventional-type Renal Cell Carcinoma

Anasuya Gunturi and David F. McDermott

Introduction

Immunotherapy was once the standard of care for patients with metastatic renal cell cancer (mRCC). However, the advent of other effective and less toxic therapies, such as vascular endothelial group factor (VEGF) and mammalian target of rapamycin (mTOR) pathway inhibitors, has led to a substantial reduction in the use of immunotherapy. Recent discoveries in tumor immunology, however, have prompted the development and study of agents that can potentially achieve durable tumor response in the absence of significant systemic toxicity. In addition, increasing awareness of the limitations of the antiangiogenic and molecularly targeted drugs alone has prompted investigations into combination therapies.

Cytokine Therapy

More than two decades ago, it was noted that removal of the primary tumor in RCC can evoke an immune response that results in spontaneous and dramatic remissions of metastases.[1] This observation soon led to investigations involving various immunotherapeutic strategies. Two cytokines, interleukin-2 (IL-2) and interferon-alpha (IFN-α), have shown antitumor activity in RCC. A Cochrane metaanalysis of randomized clinical trials showed that treatment with IFN-α was superior to controls and portended a 3.8-month survival benefit with manageable toxic effects.[2] Thus, in the absence of other effective and readily applicable treatments, the use of IFN-α became widespread and was often used as the control arm in phase 3 trials studying other therapies. With the subsequent development of various targeted agents, however, the use of IFN-α in this setting eventually decreased.

Meanwhile, the administration of high-dose (HD) IL-2 was shown to consistently produce an overall response rate of approximately 15% and durable off-treatment complete and partial responses in a minority of patients with advanced RCC.[3–5] HD IL-2 is unfortunately associated with severe toxicity including hypotension, cardiac arrhythmias, fever and chills, peripheral edema, renal failure, neurotoxicity, and rash.[6] Various alternative protocols of IL-2 have been tested to increase efficacy and minimize toxicity, including lower doses and subcutaneous or continuous delivery; however, bolus HD IL-2 was proven to be superior.[3,4] Thus, HD IL-2 therapy currently is applied only in highly selected patients who are motivated to receive this therapy and are otherwise healthy.

Recently, efforts to identify a subset of patients most likely to benefit from HD IL-2 have been undertaken. Through retrospective analysis, clinical factors such as presence of multiple metastases and presence of liver or mediastinal lymph node involvement have been shown to portend a poor response.[7] In contrast, clear-cell histology, prior nephrectomy, high performance status, and absence of bone metastases all predict a good response to HD IL-2.[8] Finally, high levels of carbonic anhydrase IX (CAIX), a transmembrane protein expressed in clear-cell RCC and thought to be a biomarker of hypoxia, were correlated with better response to IL-2 and a better prognosis overall.[9,10] These various proposed predictive models, primarily involving CAIX expression and histologic features, were tested prospectively by the Cytokine Working Group (CWG) in the SELECT trial.[11] The clinical results of this trial revealed a 25% response rate that was significantly higher than the historical experience with HD IL-2; however, the trial failed to confirm the predictive capability for CAIX staining or further improve the selection criteria for HD IL-2, thus calling into question the value of previous retrospective studies. Investigations to confirm other proposed biomarkers are needed to further understand tumor and host factors that predict for response to IL-2.

Combination of Cytokines and Antiangiogenic Therapy

In addition to single-agent cytokines, combination therapy with VEGF-targeted agents has been studied as well. Two large phase 3 trials, AVOREN and CALGB 90206, have demonstrated that in patients with mRCC, IFN plus bevacizumab has superior efficacy to IFN monotherapy, suggesting an additive effect.[12,13] The improvement, however, was only in progression-free survival (PFS), not overall survival (OS). Though these data eventually led to the US Food and Drug Administration approval of the IFN–bevacizumab combination for treatment of patients with mRCC, clarification of the relative contribution of IFN to this regimen requires a randomized trial to compare the combination with bevacizumab alone. Bevacizumab has also been combined with HD IL-2 in a CWG phase 2 trial. Investigators reported a response rate of 28% and a median PFS of 9 months; however, there were few complete responses.[14] These results suggest that these two agents may be given safely in combination and produce efficacy improvements that are additive but not synergistic.

Targeted Immunotherapy

In hopes of finding agents that would produce complete and durable responses without significant toxicities, several targeted immunotherapy approaches have been studied. Cytotoxic T-lymphocyte–associated antigen-4 (CTLA-4) is an immunoregulatory receptor expressed by T cells that interacts with the B7 molecule on antigen-presenting cells. Blocking this interaction leads to the inhibition of normally activated T cells. Two fully human anti–CTLA-4 monoclonal antibodies have been developed to date. While tremelimumab showed positive responses in metastatic melanoma in early clinical trials, it ultimately did not demonstrate superiority to standard chemotherapy in a phase 3 trial.[15] Similar investigations with tremelimumab have been limited in mRCC patients; however, another anti–CTLA-4 antibody, ipilimumab, has shown promising results. In fact, a single-institution phase 2 trial studied patients with mRCC receiving ipilimumab with a primary endpoint of response by Response Evaluation Criteria in Solid Tumors (RECIST).[16] A partial response (PR) rate of approximately 10% was noted, even in patients who had previously not responded to IL-2. Side effects included enteritis and endocrine deficiencies such as hypophysitis. Interestingly, there was a significant association between autoimmune events and tumor regression. The combination of cytokines and agents that block immune downregulation has been studied in metastatic melanoma and may offer advantage in the RCC field. For example, the combination of ipilimumab and IL-2 was studied in patients with metastatic melanoma and showed promising results.[17] Thus, it would be interesting to explore this combination in mRCC.

A critical pathway responsible for tumor-induced immune suppression in RCC is the interaction between programmed cell death 1 (PD-1) and its ligand programmed cell death ligand 1 (PD-L1), which serves to restrict the cytolytic function of tumor-infiltrating T lymphocytes.[18,19] Patients with PD-1–positive immune cells are more likely to have larger, more aggressive tumors and are at a higher risk for cancer-specific death.[20] Similarly, renal tumors that express PD-L1 behave more aggressively, leading to a shorter survival.[21] Blocking the receptor (PD-1)–ligand (PD-L1) interaction with monoclonal antibodies appears to restore the efficacy of tumor-specific T cells within the tumor microenvironment, leading to significant and sustained antitumor responses in early clinical trials.[22-24]

The first such agent was reported by Brahmer and colleagues in a phase 1 trial with nivolumab, a fully human immunoglobulin-G4 anti–PD-1 blocking antibody, in patients with selected refractory or relapsed malignancies.[22] In this trial, one complete response and two partial responses, including a patient with RCC, were observed. These results prompted investigators to include a larger cohort of RCC patients in a subsequent phase 1 trial to investigate biweekly nivolumab administration. It showed that 10 of 34 patients experienced major tumor responses and 9 other patients had stable disease that lasted at least 24 weeks.[23] Grade III or IV drug-related adverse events occurred in only 14% of the 304-patient cohort. These objective responses were also noted in patients with other malignancies such as melanoma and even non–small-cell lung cancer. Furthermore, intratumoral PD-L-1 expression seemed to correlate with tumor response to this agent. Specifically, none of the 17 patients with PD-L1–negative tumors had an objective response, while 9 of the 25 patients (36%) with PD-L1–positive tumors did. The relevance of this finding requires further exploration.

A phase 1 trial to study the efficacy of an anti–PD-L1 antibody in patients with advanced cancers including RCC was conducted as well.[24] Drug-related adverse events were generally low grade and included fatigue, infusion reactions, diarrhea, arthralgia, rash, nausea, pruritus, and headache. Several objective responses were observed, including 2 of 17 (12%) patients with RCC. Seven additional patients (41%) had stable disease that lasted at least 24 weeks. Again, similarly positive responses were noted in unexpected patient populations such as those with advanced non–small-cell lung cancer, thus making PD-L1 an exciting target for the field of oncology in general.

Combination of Targeted Immunotherapy and Antiangiogenic Therapy

While VEGF pathway–targeted therapies have significantly improved the clinical outcome for patients with advanced RCC, the development of treatment resistance leading to disease progression appears inevitable, even with continued therapy. It has been noted that elevated levels of VEGF are associated with poor prognosis in various cancers.[25] This is thought to be due to not only the angiogenic activity of VEGF but also its role in immunosuppression by inhibiting dendritic cell maturation.[26] Therefore, several investigators are testing combinations of targeted immunotherapy with agents such as sunitinib, pazopanib, or bevacizumab in hopes of enhancing their overall therapeutic effect.

In a phase 1 study, the anti–CTLA-4 antibody tremelimumab administered with sunitinib produced PRs in 9 of 21 (43%) patients with mRCC; however, a large proportion of patients unexpectedly experienced rapid-onset renal failure.[27] It may be that combinations involving VEGF pathway inhibitors and PD-1–PD-L1 pathway blockade will be better tolerated. Several such combination trials are currently underway. For example, a phase 1 trial is assessing the safety, effectiveness, and optimal dose for use of nivolumab in combination with sunitinib, pazopanib, or ipilimumab for the treatment of mRCC (NCT01472081).

Vaccines and Other Strategies

RCC continues to be an optimal disease process where novel immunotherapeutic strategies are investigated. Several years ago, it was shown that complete and partial responses could be induced in patients with refractory mRCC who underwent nonmyeloablative allogeneic stem cell transplantation.[28] Subsequent reports, however, showed less enthusiastic results. In contrast to the 53% overall response rate first reported, the response rates among the several case series that followed were highly variable, with a median response rate of only 14%. Furthermore, complete responses were rare, with most responding patients achieving only transient partial remissions and suffering subsequent disease progression.[29] Thus, the role of allogeneic stem cell transplant in RCC eventually lost favor.

Recently, there has been much interest in the development of vaccines as therapeutic agents in cancer biology. IMA901 is a therapeutic cancer vaccine developed based on multiple tumor-associated peptides (TUMAPs) known to be presented by human cancer cells. In a randomized phase 2 trial, a single dose of cyclophosphamide reduced the number of regulatory T cells and confirmed that immune responses to multiple TUMAPs were associated with longer OS.[30] This prompted a phase 3 study where the combination of IMA901 and sunitinib was investigated. Similarly, AGS-003 is a dendritic cell–based vaccine that was created by fusing patient-derived dendritic cells with autologous tumor. In a phase 2 trial, 21 patients with mRCC received AGS-003 plus sunitinib. Interim results demonstrated that median PFS was 11.2 months and median OS was 30.2 months.[31] These data led to an ongoing phase 3 study in a similar patient population.

Finally, a phase 1 trial in which patients with metastatic breast or renal cancer were treated with a vaccine prepared by fusing autologous tumor and dendritic cells showed that 5 of 13 patients with mRCC had disease stabilization, with no significant treatment-related toxicity.[32] These findings led the investigators to conduct a phase 1/2 study where 24 patients with mRCC received these vaccinations. Two of 21 evaluable patients demonstrated a partial clinical response, and 8 had stabilization of their disease.[33] Studies such as these set the foundation for future investigations of vaccine-based treatment approaches in patients with RCC.

Conclusion

An improved understanding of RCC tumor biology has led to major advances in the treatment of patients with mRCC over the past decade. Standard immunotherapy such as HD IL-2 has been shown to produce durable responses but is associated with significant toxicity. While agents that target the VEGF and mTOR pathways prolong survival, resistance eventually develops for most patients. Thus, therapies that can produce complete and durable tumor responses with an acceptable toxicity profile are much needed. Data from ongoing clinical trials suggest that targeted immunotherapy may achieve this critical unmet need. Furthermore, better patient selection and novel combination regimens may improve the efficacy of standard immunotherapy. Therefore, by drawing from our past and present cumulative experience, new successes in the application of immunotherapy in patients with RCC can be achieved.

References

1. Vogelzang NJ, Priest ER, Borden L. Spontaneous regression of histologically proved pulmonary metastases from renal cell carcinoma: a case with 5-year followup. *J Urol*. 1992;148(4):1247–1248.

2. Coppin C, Porzsolt F, Awa A, et al. Immunotherapy for advanced renal cell cancer. *Cochrane Database Syst Rev*. 2005;(1):CD001425.

3. Yang JC, Sherry RM, Steinberg SM, et al. Randomized study of high-dose and low-dose interleukin-2 in patients with metastatic renal cancer. *J Clin Oncol*. 2003;21(16):3127–3132.

4. McDermott DF, Regan MM, Clark JI, et al. Randomized phase III trial of high-dose interleukin-2 versus subcutaneous interleukin-2 and interferon in patients with metastatic renal cell carcinoma. *J Clin Oncol*. 2005;23(1):133–141.

5. Negrier S, Perol D, Ravaud A, et al. Medroxyprogesterone, interferon alfa-2a, interleukin 2, or combination of both cytokines in patients with metastatic renal carcinoma of intermediate prognosis: results of a randomized controlled trial. *Cancer*. 2007;110(11):2468–2477.

6. Dutcher J, Atkins MB, Margolin K, et al. Kidney cancer: The Cytokine Working Group experience (1986—2001), part II. Management of IL-2 toxicity and studies with other cytokines. *Med Oncol*. 2001;18(3):209–219.

7. Negrier S, Escudier B, Lasset C, et al. Recombinant human interleukin-2, recombinant human interferon alfa-2a, or both in metastatic renal-cell carcinoma. Groupe Francais d'Immunotherapie. *N Engl J Med*. 1998;338(18):1272–1278.

8. Upton MP, Parker RA, Youmans A, et al. Histologic predictors of renal cell carcinoma response to interleukin-2-based therapy. *J Immunother*. 2005;28(5):488–495.

9. Atkins M, Regan M, McDermott D, et al. Carbonic anhydrase IX expression predicts outcome of interleukin 2 therapy for renal cancer. *Clin Cancer Res*. 2005;11(10):3714–3721.

10. Bui MH, Seligson D, Han KR, et al. Carbonic anhydrase IX is an independent predictor of survival in advanced renal cell carcinoma: implications for prognosis and therapy. *Clin Cancer Res*. 2003;9(2):802–811.

11. McDermott DF, Ghebremichael MS, Signoretti S, et al. The high-dose aldesleukin (HD IL-2) "SELECT" trial in patients with metastatic renal cell carcinoma (mRCC). *J Clin Oncol*. 2010;28(15S):abstr 4514.

12. Escudier B, Pluzanska A, Koralewski P, et al. Bevacizumab plus interferon alfa-2a for treatment f metastatic renal cell carcinoma: a randomized, double-blind phase III trial. *Lancet*. 2007;370(9605):2103–2111.

13. Rini BI, Halabi S, Rosenberg JE, et al. Phase III trial of bevacizumab plus interferon alfa versus interferon alfa monotherapy in patients with metastatic renal cell carcinoma: final results of CALGB 90206. *J Clin Oncol*. 2010;28(13):2137–2143

14. Dandamudi. A phase II study of bevacizumab and high dose bolus aldesleukin (IL-2) in metastatic renal cell carcinoma patients: A Cytokine Working Group Study. *J Clin Oncol*. 2010;28(15S):abstr 5044.

15. Ribas A, Kefford R, Marshall MA, et al. Phase III randomized clinical trial comparing tremelimumab with standard-of-care chemotherapy in patients with advanced melanoma. *J Clin Oncol*. 2013;31(5):616–622.

16. Yang JC, Hughes M, Kammula U, et al. Ipilimumab (Anti-CTLA4 antibody) causes regression of metastatic renal cell cancer associated with enteritis and hypophysitis. *J Immunother*. 2007;30(8):825–830.

17. Maker AV, Phan GQ, Attia P, et al. Tumor regression and autoimmunity in patients treated with cytotoxic T lymphocyte-associated antigen 4 blockade and interleukin 2: a phase I/II study. *Ann Surg Oncol.* 2005;12(12):1005–1016.

18. Keir ME, Francisco LM, Sharpe AH. PD-1 and its ligands in T-cell immunity. *Curr Opin Immunol.* 2007;19(3):309–314.

19. Iwai Y, Ishida M, Tanaka Y, et al. Involvement of PD-L1 on tumor cells in the escape from host immune system and tumor immunotherapy by PD-L1 blockade. *Proc Natl Acad Sci USA.* 2002;99(19):12293–12297.

20. Thompson RH, Dong H, Lohse CM, et al. PD-1 is expressed by tumor-infiltrating immune cells and is associated with poor outcome for patients with renal cell carcinoma. *Clin Cancer Res.* 2007;13(6):1757–1761.

21. Thompson RH, Gillett MD, Cheville JC, et al. Costimulatory B7-H1 in renal cell carcinoma patients: indicator of tumor aggressiveness and potential therapeutic target. *Proc Natl Acad Sci USA.* 2004;101(49):17174–17179.

22. Brahmer JR, Drake CG, Wollner I, et al. Phase I study of single-agent anti-programmed death-1 (MDX-1106) in refractory solid tumors: safety, clinical activity, pharmacodynamics, and immunologic correlates. *J Clin Oncol.* 2010;28(19):3167–3175.

23. Topalian SL, Hodi FS, Brahmer JR, et al. Safety, activity, and immune correlates of anti-PD-1 antibody in cancer. *N Engl J Med.* 2012,366(26):2443–2454.

24. Brahmer JR, Tykodi SS, Chow LQ, et al. Safety and activity of anti-PD-L1 antibody in patients with advanced cancer. *N Engl J Med.* 2012; 366(26):2455–2465.

25. Poon RT, Fan ST, Wong J. Clinical implications of circulating angiogenic factors in cancer patients. *J Clin Oncol.* 2001;19(4):1207–1225.

26. Lissoni P, Malugani F, Bonfanti A, et al. Abnormally enhanced blood concentrations of vascular endothelial growth factor (VEGF) in metastatic cancer patients and their relation to circulating dendritic cells, IL-12 and endothelin-1. *J Biol Regul Homeost Agents.* 2001;15(2):140–144.

27. Rini BI, Stein M, Shannon P, et al. Phase I dose-escalation trial of tremelimumab plus sunitinib in patients with metastatic renal cell carcinoma. *Cancer.* 2011; 117(4):758–767.

28. Childs R, Chernoff A, Contentin N, et al. Regression of metastatic renal-cell carcinoma after nonmyeloablative allogeneic peripheral-blood stem-cell transplantation. *N Engl J Med.* 2000;343(11):750–758.

29. Tykodi SS, Sandmaier BM, Warren EH, et al. Allogeneic hematopoietic cell transplantation for renal cell carcinoma: ten years after. *Expert Opin Biol Ther.* 2011;11(6):763–773.

30. Walter S, Weinschenk T, Stenzl A, et al. Multipeptide immune response to cancer vaccine IMA901 after single-dose cyclophosphamide associates with longer patient survival. *Nature Medicine.* 2012;18(8):1254–1261.

31. Amin A. Prolonged survival with personalized immunotherapy (AGS-003) in combination with sunitinib in unfavorable risk metastatic RCC (mRCC) Presented at: Genitourinary Cancers Symposium; February 14–16, 2013; Orlando, FL.

32. Avigan D, Vasir B, Gong J, et al. Fusion cell vaccination of patients with metastatic breast and renal cancer induces immunological and clinical responses. *Clin Cancer Res.* 2004;10(14):4699–4708.

33. Avigan DE, Vasir B, George DJ, et al. Phase I/II study of vaccination with electrofused allogeneic dendritic cells/autologous tumor-derived cells in patients with stage IV renal cell carcinoma. *J Immunother.* 2007;30(7):749–761.

Chapter 10

Targeted Therapies for Metastatic Conventional-type Renal Cell Carcinoma

Tim Eisen and Ferdinandos Skoulidis

Introduction

Conventional-type renal cell carcinoma (RCC) is resistant to chemotherapy. Immunotherapy with either interferon-alpha (IFN-α) or interleukin-2 (IL-2) constituted the mainstay of systemic therapy for this malignant disease until less than a decade ago.

Since that time, molecularly targeted therapies have revolutionized the management and altered the natural history of metastatic RCC (mRCC). Since the original report of the pivotal TARGET trial (treatment approaches in renal cancer global evaluation trial) in 2005, four small-molecule receptor tyrosine kinase (RTK) inhibitors—sorafenib, sunitinib, pazopanib, and axitinib—and the anti-vascular endothelial growth factor (VEGF) monoclonal antibody bevacizumab (in combination with IFN-α) have received regulatory approval for this disease. More recently temsirolimus and everolimus, two inhibitors of mammalian target of rapamycin (mTOR), have further expanded our therapeutic armamentarium for this disease.

With the exception of temsirolimus, the only agent with a demonstrated overall survival (OS) advantage in a pivotal phase 3 trial, all agents have attained regulatory approval on the basis of prolongation of progression-free survival (PFS) compared with either cytokine-based therapy (IFN-α) or placebo. The expanded availability of accessible effective therapies since the original approval of sorafenib in 2005, coupled with high rates of crossover in recent clinical trials of novel VEGF and mTOR inhibitors, and administration of multiple subsequent lines of treatment "off trial" have confounded the potential impact of individual agents on OS. Nonetheless, it is clear that patients with mRCC who receive modern-era sequential targeted therapy live longer, with median OS >29 months in recently reported clinical trials compared with the historical control of 13 months in the immunotherapy era. A treatment algorithm that is supported by current best evidence is presented in Table 10.1.

Table 10.1 Algorithm for Systemic Therapy of Metastatic Clear-Cell Renal Cell Carcinoma Based on Current Best Evidence

Setting		Standard	Option
First line	Favorable prognostic group	Pazopanib Sunitinib Bevacizumab + IFN-α	High-dose interleukin-2 Sorafenib
	Intermediate prognostic group	Pazopanib Sunitinib Bevacizumab + IFN-α	Sorafenib
	Poor prognostic group	Temsirolimus	Sunitinib
Second line	Prior cytokine-based therapy	Axitinib Sorafenib Pazopanib	Sunitinib
	One prior VEGF-pathway–directed therapy	Everolimus Axitinib	Sorafenib
Third line	Two prior VEGF-pathway–directed agents	Everolimus	Clinical trial
	Prior VEGF-pathway and mTOR inhibitor		Tyrosine kinase inhibitor Clinical trial

Data are current as of March 2014
IFN-α, interferon-alpha; VEGF, vascular endothelial growth factor.

First-line Therapy of Treatment-Naïve Patients

An important challenge in the initial management of mRCC is to define the optimal time for initiation of systemic therapy. A small subset (5%–10%) of RCCs run an indolent clinical course that is characterized by slowly progressive metastatic disease over a number of years.[1] Therefore, assessment of tumor growth kinetics with serial imaging (eg, every 2–3 months) during a planned period of observation constitutes a valid therapeutic approach for patients with favorable- and intermediate-risk disease, low tumor burden, and no critical lesions and may help identify a subgroup of patients in whom systemic therapy can be safely deferred.[2] Following initial surveillance, systemic therapy should be recommended in the event of disease-related symptoms or significant radiological progression or when patients find it difficult to cope with the psychological burden of ongoing observation.

As of April 2014, five targeted agents had received regulatory approval in the United States and Europe for the first-line treatment of patients with metastatic clear-cell renal cell carcinoma (ccRCC). Pivotal phase 3 and selected phase 2 trials of these agents in the first-line treatment of ccRCC are listed in Table 10.2.

Table 10.2 Phase 3 and Selected Randomized Phase 2 Trials of Targeted Agents in the First-line Treatment of Metastatic Clear-Cell Renal Cell Carcinoma

Trial and Reference	Line of Treatment	Treatment Arms	Number of Patients	Patient Population	Median Progression-Free Survival (months)	Median Overall Survival (months)	Objective Response Rate (%)
NCT00083889: 3, 4	First	Sunitinib vs INF-α	750	Treatment naïve • Clear-cell histology • PS 0-1 • 90% prior nephrectomy • MSKCC risk group: - 36% favorable - 57.4% intermediate - 6.6% unknown	11.0* 5.0*	26.4^{NS} 21.8^{NS}	31* 6*

(Continued)

Table 10.2 (Continued)

Trial and Reference	Line of Treatment	Treatment Arms	Number of Patients	Patient Population	Median Progression-Free Survival (months)	Median Overall Survival (months)	Objective Response Rate (%)

VEG105192: 5, 6	First/second (after cytokine failure)	Pazopanib vs placebo	435 (2:1)	Treatment naïve or following cytokine failure
				• Clear-cell or predominantly clear-cell histology
				• Metastatic/locally advanced
				• PS 0–1
				• 88.5% prior nephrectomy
				• MSKCC risk group:
				  - 39.1% favorable
				  - 54.3% intermediate
				  - 3.2% poor
				  - 3.4% unknown
				Subgroup analysis:
				  - Treatment naïve
				  - Cytokine pretreated
					9.2*
					
					4.2*
					
					11.1* vs 2.8*
					7.4* vs 4.2*
						22.9^{NS}
						
						20.5^{NS}
							30*
							
							3*
							
							32* vs 4*
							29* vs 3*

COMPARZ: 7	First	Sunitinib vs pazopanib	1110	Treatment naïve • Clear-cell histology • KPS≥70% • 83% prior nephrectomy • MSKCC risk group: - 27.3% favorable - 58.6% intermediate - 10.7% poor - 3.4% unknown	9.5^{NS} 8.4^{NS}	29.3^{NS} 28.4^{NS}	24 31
AVOREN: 9,10	First	Bevacizumab + INF-α-2a vs INF-α-2a	649	Treatment naïve • Predominantly (>50%) clear-cell histology • Metastatic • KPS ≥70% • 100% prior nephrectomy • MSKCC risk group: - 27.7% favorable - 56% intermediate - 8.3% poor - 8% unknown	10.2^{*} 5.4^{*}	23.3^{NS} 21.3^{NS}	31^{*} 13^{*}

(Continued)

Table 10.2 (Continued)

Trial and Reference	Line of Treatment	Treatment Arms	Number of Patients	Patient Population	Median Progression-Free Survival (months)	Median Overall Survival (months)	Objective Response Rate (%)

CALGB 90206: 11, 12	First	Bevacizumab+ IFN-α-2b vs IFN-α-2b	732	Treatment naïve
				• Clear-cell histology component present
				• Metastatic
				• KPS ≥70%
				• 85% prior nephrectomy
				• MSKCC risk group:
				  - 26% favorable
				  - 64% intermediate
				  - 10% poor
					8.5*
					
					5.2*
						18.3^{NS}
						
						17.4^{NS}
							25.5*
							
							13.1*
							(investigator assessed)

Global ARCC: 18	First	Temsirolimus vs IFN-α vs temsirolimus +IFN-α	626	Treatment naïve
				• Clear-cell (80%) and non–clear-cell histology (20%)
				• Stage IV or recurrent disease
				• KPS ≤70% (82.4%)
				• 67% prior nephrectomy
				• MSKCC risk group:
				  - 74% poor
				  - 26% intermediate
					5.5
					
					3.1
					
					4.7
						10.9*
						
						7.3*
						
						8.4^{NS}
							8.6
							
							4.8
							
							8.1

Trial	Line	Treatment	N	Patient characteristics			

TIVO-1: 16	First	Tivozanib vs sorafenib	517	Treatment naive or one prior therapy (excluding vascular endothelial growth factor– and mammalian target of rapamycin–pathway inhibitors)
				• Clear-cell histology
				• Metastatic
				• Predominant enrollment in Central/Eastern Europe
				• PS 0-1
				• 100% prior nephrectomy
				• MSKCC risk group:
				  - 30.4% favorable
				  - 64.4% intermediate
				  - 5.2% poor
					11.9*
					
					9.1*
						28.8^{NS}
						
						29.3^{NS}
							33.1*
							
							23.3*

AGILE 1051: 17	First	Axitinib vs sorafenib	288 (2:1)	Treatment naive
				• Clear-cell histology
				• Metastatic
				• 51% Eastern European origin
				• PS 0-1
				• 86.5% prior nephrectomy
				• MSKCC risk group:
				  - 51% favorable
				  - 43.1% intermediate
				  - 3.1% poor
				  - 2.8 unknown
					10.1^{NS}
					
					6.5^{NS}
						NA
						
						NA
							32*
							
							15*

(Continued)

Table 10.2 (Continued)

Trial and Reference	Line of Treatment	Treatment Arms	Number of Patients	Patient Population	Median Progression-Free Survival (months)	Median Overall Survival (months)	Objective Response Rate (%)

INTORACT (investigation of torisel and avastin combination therapy): 20	First	Bevacizumab + temsirolimus vs bevacizumab + IFN	791	Treatment naive
				• Predominantly clear-cell histology
				• Metastatic
				• KPS ≥70%
				• 85.5% prior nephrectomy
				• MSKCC risk group:
				  - 30% favorable
				  - 59% intermediate
				  - 11% poor
					9.1[NS]
					
					9.3[NS]
						25.8[NS]
						
						25.5[NS]
							27[NS]
							
							27.4[NS]

RECORD-2: 21 (randomized phase 2)	First	Bevacizumab + everolimus vs bevacizumab + IFN-α-2a	365	Treatment naive
				• Clear-cell histology
				• Metastatic
				• KPS ≥70%
				• 100% prior nephrectomy
				• MSKCC risk group:
				  - 36% favorable
				  - 57% intermediate
				  - 7% poor
					9.3[NS]
					
					10.02[NS]
						NA
						
						25.86
							26.9[NS]
							
							27.9[NS]

Trial	Line	Treatment	N	Patient characteristics	PFS (months)	OS	Response (%)
TORAVA (torisel and avastin trial): 22	First	Bevacizumab + temsirolimus vs sunitinib vs bevacizumab + IFN-α-2a	171 (2:1:1)	No prior systemic therapy • Any histological subtype except for papillary (96% clear cell) • 87% prior nephrectomy • PS ≤2 • MSKCC risk group: - 33.5% favorable - 52.6% intermediate - 13.8% poor	8.2^{NS} 8.2^{NS} 16.8^{NS}	$37\%^{NS}$(35m) $55\%^{NS}$(35m) $62\%^{*}$(35m)	27 29 43
BeST (randomized phase 2): 23	First	Bevacizumab vs bevacizumab + temsirolimus vs bevacizumab + sorafenib vs sorafenib + temsirolimus	361	Treatment naïve or cytokine/vaccine pretreated (one prior line of therapy) • Predominantly (≥75%) clear-cell histology • 87% prior nephrectomy • MSKCC risk group: - 32% favorable - 40% intermediate - 28% poor	8.7^{NS} 7.3^{NS} 11.3^{NS} 7.7^{NS}	NA NA NA NA	12^{*} 29^{*} 30^{*} 26^{*}

INF-α, interferon-alpha; PS, performance status; KPS, Karnofsky performance status; NA, not applicable; MSKCC, Memorial Sloan-Kettering Cancer Center; NS, not statistically significant
* Denotes statistical significance at the p≤0.05 level.

Sunitinib is an orally bioavailable small-molecule tyrosine kinase inhibitor (TKI) with low nanomolar potency against a number of angiogenic receptor tyrosine kinases, including VEGFR-1, -2, and -3 (vascular endothelial growth factor receptor) and PDGFR-α and -β (platelet-derived growth factor receptor). Inhibitory activity has also been demonstrated against the FLT3 kinase (feline McDonough sarcoma–related tyrosine kinase), as well as c-KIT (v-Kit Hardy–Zuckerman 4 feline sarcoma viral oncogene homolog), colony-stimulating factor-1R, and the RET (rearranged during transfection proto-oncogene) kinase. The US Food and Drug Administration (FDA) approved sunitinib in January 2006 for the treatment of patients with advanced RCC and it represents the most widely prescribed first-line targeted therapy for treatment-naïve patients in the Western world and a standard of care for this disease. It is administered orally at a dose of 50 mg once daily for 4 weeks followed by a 2-week break ("4/2 schedule"). Sunitinib is metabolized predominantly by the cytochrome P450-3A4 pathway (CYP3A4) in hepatic microsomes. Therefore, concomitant administration of potent CYP3A4 inducers (eg, rifampicin) or inhibitors (eg, clarithromycin) may significantly affect sunitinib plasma exposure and should be avoided. Commonly prescribed drugs that can induce or inhibit the P450-3A4 pathway are listed in Table 10.3.

The pivotal NCT00083889 phase 3 trial randomized 750 previously untreated patients with metastatic ccRCC to receive either sunitinib 50 mg daily orally on a 4/2 schedule or IFN-α at a dose of 9 MU subcutaneously three times a week.[3] At the second preplanned interim analysis, the trial met its primary endpoint by demonstrating a statistically significant and clinically meaningful prolongation of median PFS from 5 months for the IFN arm to 11 months for the sunitinib arm, corresponding to a 58% reduction in the risk of progression or death (hazard ratio [HR], 0.42; 95% confidence interval [CI], 0.32–0.54; $P<0.001$). Evidence for antitumor efficacy was further substantiated by a 31% objective response rate compared with 6% for IFN. At the time of the final OS analysis, there was a strong trend toward improved OS with sunitinib (median OS, 26.4 months) compared with IFN (median OS, 21.8 months; HR for death, 0.821; 95% CI, 0.673–1.001; $P=0.051$).[4]

Pazopanib is an orally active small-molecule TKI. Its activity in patients with mRCC was established in the VEG105192 phase 3 clinical trial.[5,6] In this trial, 435 patients with ccRCC (90%) or predominantly ccRCC (10%) were randomized on a 2:1 ratio to receive either pazopanib 800 mg orally once daily continuously or placebo. The trial enrolled both treatment-naïve (53%) and cytokine-pretreated patients (47%). Pazopanib resulted in a significant PFS benefit compared with placebo (9.2 months versus 4.2 months; HR, 0.46; 95% CI, 0.34–0.62; $P<0.0001$). The benefit was even more pronounced in the subpopulation of treatment-naïve patients (11.1 months versus 2.8 months; HR, 0.40; 95% CI, 0.27–0.60; $P<0.0001$) and numerically approximate to the median PFS previously reported with sunitinib. The objective response rate reported in the pazopanib arm was 30%.

The FDA approved pazopanib for the treatment of patients with advanced RCC in October 2009. The results of a head-to-head comparison between sunitinib and pazopanib were eagerly anticipated. The COMPARZ trial

Table 10.3 Drugs That Affect Hepatic CYP3A4

CYP3A4 Inhibitors*

Strong inhibitors:	Moderate inhibitors:
Clarithromycin	Aprepitant
Telithromycin	Ciprofloxacin
Indinavir	Erythromycin
Ritonavir	Fluconazole
Lopinavir/ritonavir	Diltiazem
Saquinavir	Verapamil
Nelfinavir	Amprenavir
Telaprevir	Atazanavir
Boceprevir	Fosamprenavir
Itraconazole	Darunavir/ritonavir
Ketoconazole	Grapefruit juice
Voriconazole	
Posaconazole	
Nefazodone	
Mibefradil	
Conivaptan	
Grapefruit juice	

CYP3A4 Inducers†

Carbamazepine
Phenytoin
Rifampin/Rifampicin
Avasimibe
Efavirenz
Etravirine
Bosentan
Modafinil
Nafcillin
Dexamethasone
Prednisolone
St. John's wort

*May increase levels of tyrosine kinase inhibitor or mammalian target of rapamycin inhibitor.
†May decrease levels of tyrosine kinase inhibitor or mammalian target of rapamycin inhibitor.

(comparing the efficacy, safety, and tolerability of pazopanib versus sunitinib) was designed as a noninferiority trial in which 1110 treatment-naïve patients with advanced/metastatic ccRCC were randomized on a 1:1 ratio to receive either sunitinib or pazopanib.[7] The COMPARZ trial demonstrated a median PFS of 8.4 months for pazopanib and 9.5 months for sunitinib (HR, 1.047; 95% CI, 0.898–1.220). With the noninferiority margin set at 1.25, the trial met its primary endpoint in the main intention-to-treat analysis, thus demonstrating noninferiority of pazopanib compared with sunitinib for PFS. OS was also similar (HR for death with pazopanib, 0.91; 95% CI, 0.76–1.08). The quality-of-life (QoL) assessment favored pazopanib, although concerns have been raised that the timing of QoL assessments may have disadvantaged sunitinib in this trial.

Patient preference for pazopanib or sunitinib was the primary endpoint of the randomized phase 2 PISCES trial (pazopanib versus sunitinib patient preference study in treatment-naïve metastatic renal cell carcinoma).[8] One hundred and sixty-eight patients with mRCC (90% clear-cell) were randomized to either initial pazopanib (10 weeks, continuous dosing) followed by subsequent sunitinib (10 weeks, 4/2 schedule) or the opposite schedule of sunitinib followed by pazopanib. At the end of the 22-week treatment period, 70% of patients indicated that they preferred pazopanib over sunitinib. Less fatigue and improved QoL were the main reasons cited for patient preference for pazopanib.

Based on the results of the COMPARZ and PISCES clinical trials, pazopanib is increasingly considered the preferred first-line angiogenesis inhibitor.

Targeting soluble VEGF with monoclonal antibodies is an alternative anti-angiogenic strategy. Bevacizumab is a recombinant humanized anti–VEGF-A monoclonal antibody that was FDA approved in July 2009 for the treatment of advanced RCC in combination with IFN-α. Regulatory approval was based on the results of two large phase 3 clinical trials: the European AVOREN (avastin and roferon in renal cell carcinoma) and the US-led CALGB (Cancer and Leukemia Group B) 90206.[9–12] Both trials reported significantly prolonged median PFS in the bevacizumab–IFN-α arm (AVOREN: 10.2 months versus 5.4 months in the placebo–IFN-α arm; HR, 0.63; 95% CI, 0.52–0.75; $P=0.0001$; and CALGB 90206: 8.5 months versus 5.2 months in the INF-α arm; adjusted HR, 0.71; 95% CI, 0.61–0.83; $P<0.0001$).

Sorafenib, a multitargeted TKI, was the first targeted agent to receive regulatory approval for the treatment of advanced RCC in December 2005. The registration phase 3 trial of sorafenib was conducted in a patient population previously treated with cytokines (IFN-α, IL-2, or both), a standard first-line treatment option at the time.[13,14] Until 2012, no large phase 3 clinical trial of sorafenib in previously untreated patients had reported results; however, randomized phase 2 trials yielded PFS ranging from 5.7 months to 9.0 months in the first-line setting.[15] More recently, the TIVO-1 (tivozanib versus sorafenib in first-line advanced RCC) and AGILE 1051 (axitinib [AG-013736] for the treatment of metastatic RCC) phase 3 clinical trials reported PFS of 9.1 months and 6.5 months, respectively, in the sorafenib (active control) arm.[16,17] Based on current best evidence, sorafenib is not considered a standard first-line therapy for advanced RCC, although some clinicians use it in patients with significant cardiovascular or other comorbidities.

The clinical efficacy of axitinib, a highly potent and selective TKI, was compared with that of sorafenib in the AGILE 1051 multicenter randomized phase 3 clinical trial.[17] Two hundred and eighty-eight treatment-naïve patients with metastatic ccRCC, predominantly from Eastern Europe and Asia, were randomized on a 2:1 allocation ratio to axitinib at a dose of 5 mg twice daily orally or sorafenib 400 mg twice daily orally. Although median PFS was prolonged by 3.6 months in patients receiving axitinib (10.1 months versus 6.5 months), the trial failed to achieve its primary endpoint statistically. Consequently, use of axitinib in the first-line setting cannot be recommended based on currently available evidence.

On the basis of data from the Global ARCC (advanced RCC) trial, temsirolimus is licensed for patients with metastatic, poor-risk RCC and is widely used in the United States for this indication.[18] In Europe, a substantial fraction of patients with poor-risk disease receive sunitinib on the basis of subgroup analysis from the pivotal trial (NCT00083889) and data from the sunitinib expanded-access program.[3,19]

Combination regimens consisting of either two VEGF pathway inhibitors (vertical inhibition) or a VEGF and mTOR inhibitor (horizontal inhibition) have also been evaluated in clinical trials but cannot be recommended on the basis of current best evidence (Table 10.3).[20–23]

Second-line Therapy Following Cytokine Failure

Two agents, sorafenib and axitinib, are recommended on the basis of level 1 evidence following failure of cytokine-based therapy.

In the TARGET trial, 903 patients with ccRCC who had progressed after one previous line of non-VEGF pathway-based therapy (mostly cytokine-based) were randomized to receive either sorafenib or placebo.[13,14] Sorafenib conferred significant improvement in median PFS from 2.8 months to 5.5 months (HR, 0.44; 95% CI, 0.35–0.55; $P<0.01$) and was associated with a 10% objective response rate compared with 2% in the placebo arm ($P<0.001$). The activity of axitinib in the second-line setting following cytokine failure was established in the multicenter AXIS (axitinib [AG013736] as second-line therapy for mRCC) randomized phase 3 clinical trial.[24,25] Seven hundred and twenty-three patients were stratified according to performance status (0 versus 1) and previous first-line therapy and subsequently randomized to axitinib or sorafenib. Whereas the trial met its primary endpoint by demonstrating a significant prolongation of median PFS (per independent radiology review) in the axitinib arm regardless of prior therapy (6.7 months versus 4.7 months; HR, 0.665; 95% CI, 0.544–0.812; one-sided $P<0.0001$), the effect of axitinib was most impressive in the subgroup of cytokine-pretreated patients, where it conferred a 12.1-month median PFS compared with 6.5 months in the sorafenib arm. Subgroup analysis of the VEG105192 trial revealed that pazopanib also has activity in patients with progressive disease following cytokine-based therapy (median PFS 7.4 months in the pazopanib arm compared with 4.2 months with placebo; HR, 0.54; 95% CI, 0.35–0.94; $P<0.001$).[5] Sunitinib also demonstrated activity in this setting, although the clinical evidence supporting its use in this context is less robust.[15] Table 10.4 summarizes the key phase 3 trials of targeted therapies in the second-line setting.

Second-line Therapy Following Failure of a Vascular Endothelial Growth Factor Pathway–Targeted Agent

Two therapeutic strategies can be implemented for patients who develop progressive disease following VEGF–pathway-targeted therapy: treatment

Table 10.4 Phase 3 Clinical Trials of Targeted Agents in the Second-line Treatment of Metastatic Clear-Cell Renal Cell Carcinoma

Trial	Line of Treatment	Treatment Arms	Number of Patients	Patient Population	Median Progression-Free Survival (months)	Median Overall Survival (months)	Objective Response Rate (%)

TARGET: 13, 14	First; after one systemic, non-VEGF pathway-targeted therapy	Sorafenib vs placebo	903	Progression after one systemic therapy within previous 8 months; VEGF pathway inhibitors excluded
				• Clear-cell histology (99%)
				• Metastatic
				• 82% prior cytokine-based therapy
				• PS 0-1
				• 93.4% prior nephrectomy
				• MSKCC risk group:
				  - 51% favorable
				  - 49% intermediate
					5.5*
					
					2.8*
						17.8*[NS]
						
						15.2*[NS]
							10*
							
							2*

| VEGF105192; 5, 6 | First/second; after cytokine failure | Pazopanib vs placebo | 435 (202 cytokine-pretreated) 2:1 | Treatment naïve or following cytokine failure
• Clear-cell or predominantly clear-cell histology
• Metastatic/locally advanced
• PS 0-1
• 88.5% prior nephrectomy
• MSKCC risk group:
  - 39.1% favorable
  - 54.3% intermediate
  - 3.2% poor
  - 3.4% unknown | 7.4* (cytokine-pretreated)

4.2* (cytokine-pre-treated) | NA

NA | 29* (cytokine-pretreated)

3* (cytokine-pretreated) |

(Continued)

Table 10.4 (Continued)

Trial	Line of Treatment	Treatment Arms	Number of Patients	Patient Population	Median Progression-Free Survival (months)	Median Overall Survival (months)	Objective Response Rate (%)
AXIS: 24, 25	Second: following sunitinib or cytokine-based or bevacizumab + IFN-α or temsirolimus	Axitinib vs sorafenib	723	Failure of one previous systemic first-line regimen: • > 54% sunitinib • > 35% cytokine based • > 8% bevacizumab • > 3% temsirolimus • Clear-cell component on histological or cytological exam • PS 0-1 • 91% prior nephrectomy • MSKCC risk group(3-factor): - 27.8% favorable - 36.5% intermediate - 32.9% poor - 2.8% unknown • Heng risk score: - 20% favorable - 63.8% intermediate - 9.8% poor - 6.4% unknown	6.7* (12.1* in cytokine-pretreated and 4.8* in sunitinib pretreated) 4.7* (6.5* in cytokine pretreated and 3.4* in sunitinib-pretreated)	20.1^{NS} (29.4-prior cytokines, 15.2-prior sunitinib) 19.2^{NS} (27.8-prior cytokines, 18-prior sunitinib)	19.4* 9.4*

Trial	Setting	Treatment	N (randomization)	Patient characteristics	PFS (mo)	OS (mo)	ORR (%)
RECORD-1: 26, 27	Second; following failure of VEGF-targeted therapy	Everolimus vs placebo	410 (2:1)	- Progression within 6 months of sunitinib (45%), sorafenib (29%), or both (26%); prior therapy with cytokines (51% IFN) and/or bevacizumab (9%) allowed • Clear-cell component • KPS ≥70 • 96% prior nephrectomy • MSKCC risk group (3-factor) - 29% favorable - 56% intermediate - 15% poor	4.9* 1.9*	14.8^{NS} 14.4^{NS}	1.8 0
INTORSECT	Second; after sunitinib failure	Temsirolimus vs sorafenib	512	Following failure of first-line therapy with sunitinib • Clear-cell (82.4%) and non-clear-cell (17.6%) histology • PS 0-1 • 86% prior nephrectomy • MSKCC risk group (3-factor) - 18.4% favorable - 69.3% intermediate - 12.3% poor	4.3^{NS} 3.9^{NS}	12.3* 16.6*	8 8

INF-α, interferon-alpha; PS, performance status; NA, not applicable; KPS, Karnofsky performance status; MSKCC, Memorial Sloan-Kettering Cancer Center;, not statistically significant; VEGF, vascular endothelial growth factor.
*Denotes statistical significance at p≤0.05 level.

with a different VEGF pathway inhibitor or pathway "switch" to an mTOR inhibitor.

Proponents of the first approach draw support from the results of the aforementioned AXIS trial.[24,25] In the subgroup of patients who developed progressive disease following upfront treatment with sunitinib, the use of axitinib resulted in a median PFS of 4.8 months compared with 3.4 months for patients who received sorafenib (HR, 0.741; 95% CI, 0.573–0.958; $P=0.0107$). More recently, the INTORSECT (investigating TORISEL as second-line therapy) trial demonstrated an OS benefit in favor of sorafenib (median OS 16.6 months) compared to temsirolimus (median OS 12.3 months) in patients who had progressed on sunitinib (HR = 1.31; 95% CI, 1.05-1.63; $P = 0.01$)[26].

The earlier RECORD-1 (RCC treatment with oral RAD001 given daily) phase 3 trial established the use of the mTOR inhibitor everolimus as a standard of care following failure of upfront TKI therapy.[27,28] Four hundred and ten patients were randomized on a 2:1 ratio to receive everolimus at a dose of 10 mg once daily orally or matched placebo. Of note, 26% of patients in this trial had previously been exposed to both sunitinib and sorafenib and were thus receiving treatment with everolimus or placebo in the third-line setting. Median PFS for the whole population was 4.9 months in the everolimus arm, compared with 1.9 months in the placebo arm (HR, 0.33; $P < 0.001$). For sunitinib-only pretreated patients, median PFS was 4.6 months for everolimus and 1.8 months for placebo (HR, 0.30; $P<0.0001$). Finally, for the subgroup of patients with progressive disease following two previous TKIs, median PFS was 4.0 months in the everolimus arm, indicating activity for this drug in the third-line setting, albeit less pronounced compared with its use following failure of a single TKI.

Third-line Therapy

Following failure of second-line therapy, enrollment into clinical trials is recommended. Patients who have received prior cytokine-based therapy and one VEGF-pathway inhibitor or two prior VEGF-pathway inhibitors can be considered for everolimus, based on subgroup analyses of the RECORD-1 clinical trial.[27,28] Patients previously exposed to both VEGF and mTOR–targeted therapy can be considered for rechallenge with a TKI.

References

1. Rini BI, Campbell SC, Escudier B. Renal cell carcinoma. *Lancet*. 2009;373(9669):1119–1132.

2. Fisher R, Pender A, Thillai K, et al. Observation as a treatment strategy for advanced renal cell carcinoma-a call for prospective validation. *Front Oncol*. 2012;2(155): 1–2.

3. Motzer RJ, Hutson TE, Tomczak P, et al. Sunitinib versus interferon alfa in metastatic renal-cell carcinoma. *N Engl J Med*. 2007;356(2):115–124.

4. Motzer RJ, Hutson TE, Tomczak P, et al. Overall survival and updated results for sunitinib compared with interferon alfa in patients with metastatic renal cell carcinoma. *J Clin Oncol*. 2009;27(22):3584–3590.

5. Sternberg CN, Davis ID, Mardiak J, et al. Pazopanib in locally advanced or metastatic renal cell carcinoma: results of a randomized phase III trial. *J Clin Oncol.* 2010;28(6):1061–1068.

6. Sternberg CN, Hawkins RE, Wagstaff J,et al. A randomised, double-blind phase III study of pazopanib in patients with advanced and/or metastatic renal cell carcinoma: final overall survival results and safety update. *Eur J Cancer.* 2013;49(6):1287–1296.

7. Motzer RJ, Hutson TE, Cella D, et al. Pazopanib versus sunitinib in metastatic renal-cell carcinoma. *N Engl J Med.*2013;369(8):722–731.

8. Escudier B, Porta C, Bono P, et al. Randomized, controlled, double-blind, cross-over trial assessing treatment preference for pazopanib versus sunitinib in patients with metastatic renal cell carcinoma: PISCES study. *J Clin Oncol.* 2014 [Epub ahead of print].

9. Escudier B, Pluzanska A, Koralewski P, et al. Bevacizumab plus interferon alfa-2a for treatment of metastatic renal cell carcinoma: a randomised, double-blind phase III trial. *Lancet.* 2007;370(9605):2103–2111.

10. Escudier B, Bellmunt J, Negrier S, et al. Phase III trial of bevacizumab plus interferon alfa-2a in patients with metastatic renal cell carcinoma (AVOREN): final analysis of overall survival. *J Clin Oncol.* 2010;28(13):2144–2150.

11. Rini BI, Halabi S, Rosenberg JE, et al. Bevacizumab plus interferon alfa compared with interferon alfa monotherapy in patients with metastatic renal cell carcinoma: CALGB 90206. *J Clin Oncol.* 2008;26(33):5422–5428.

12. Rini BI, Halabi S, Rosenberg JE, et al. Phase III trial of bevacizumab plus interferon alfa versus interferon alfa monotherapy in patients with metastatic renal cell carcinoma: final results of CALGB 90206. *J Clin Oncol.* 2010;28(13):2137–2143.

13. Escudier B, Eisen T, Stadler WM, et al. Sorafenib in advanced clear-cell renal-cell carcinoma. *N Engl J Med.* 2007;356(2):125–134.

14. Escudier B, Eisen T, Stadler WM, et al. Sorafenib for treatment of renal cell carcinoma: Final efficacy and safety results of the phase III treatment approaches in renal cancer global evaluation trial. *J Clin Oncol.* 2009;27(20):3312–3318.

15. Escudier B, Szczylik C, Porta C, Gore M. Treatment selection in metastatic renal cell carcinoma: expert consensus. *Nat Rev Clin Oncol.* 2012;9(6):327–337.

16. Motzer RJ, Nosov D, Eisen T, et al. Tivozanib versus sorafenib as initial targeted therapy for patients with metastatic renal cell carcinoma: results from a phase III trial. *J Clin Oncol.* 2013;31(30):3791–3799.

17. Hutson TE, Lesovoy V, Al-Shukri S, et al. Axitinib versus sorafenib as first-line therapy in patients with metastatic renal-cell carcinoma: a randomised open-label phase 3 trial. *Lancet Oncol.* 2013;14(13):1287–1294.

18. Hudes G, Carducci M, Tomczak P, et al. Temsirolimus, interferon alfa, or both for advanced renal-cell carcinoma. *N Engl J Med.* 2007;356(22):2271–2281.

19. Gore ME, Szczylik C, Porta C, et al. Safety and efficacy of sunitinib for metastatic renal-cell carcinoma: an expanded-access trial. *Lancet Oncol.* 2009;10(8):757–763.

20. Rini BI, Bellmunt J, Clancy J, Wang K, Niethammer AG, Hariharan S, Escudier B. Randomized Phase III Trial of Temsirolimus and Bevacizumab Versus Interferon Alfa and Bevacizumab in Metastatic Renal Cell Carcinoma: INTORACT Trial. *J Clin Oncol.* 2014;32(8):752-759.

21. Ravaud A, Barrios C, Anak O, et al. Randomized phase II study of first-line everolimus (EVE) + bevacizumab (BEV) versus interferon-alfa-2a (IFN) + BEV

in patients (PTS) with metastatic renal cell carcinoma (MRCC): RECORD-2. *Ann Oncol.* 2012;23(suppl9; abstr 783).

22. Negrier S, Gravis G, Perol D, et al. Temsirolimus and bevacizumab, or sunitinib, or interferon alfa and bevacizumab for patients with advanced renal cell carcinoma (TORAVA): a randomised phase 2 trial. *Lancet Oncol.* 2011;12(7):673–680.

23. Flaherty K. A randomized phase II study of VEGF, RAF kinase and mTOR combination targeted therapy with bevacizumab, sorafenib and temsirolimus in advanced renal cell carcinoma. Paper presented at:11th International Kidney Cancer Symposium; October 2012; Chicago IL.

24. Rini BI, Escudier B, Tomczak P, et al. Comparative effectiveness of axitinib versus sorafenib in advanced renal cell carcinoma (AXIS): a randomised phase 3 trial. *Lancet.* 2011;378(9807):1931–1939.

25. Motzer RJ, Escudier B, Tomczak P, et al. Axitinib versus sorafenib as second-line treatment for advanced renal cell carcinoma: overall survival analysis and updated results from a randomised phase 3 trial. *Lancet Oncol.* 2013;14(6):552–562.

26. Hutson TE, Escudier B, Esteban E, et al. Randomized Phase III Trial of Temsirolimus Versus Sorafenib As Second-Line Therapy After Sunitinib in Patients With Metastatic Renal Cell Carcinoma. *J Clin Oncol.* 2014;32(8):760–767.

27. Motzer RJ, Escudier B, Oudard S, et al. Efficacy of everolimus in advanced renal cell carcinoma: a double-blind, randomised, placebo-controlled phase III trial. *Lancet.* 2008;372(9637):449–456.

28. Motzer RJ, Escudier B, Oudard S, et al. Phase 3 trial of everolimus for metastatic renal cell carcinoma: final results and analysis of prognostic factors. *Cancer.* 2010;116(18):4256–4265.

Chapter 11

Systemic Therapies for Metastatic Renal Cell Carcinoma of Variant Histology

Sumanta K. Pal and Toni K. Choueiri

Introduction

It is unclear whether or not benefits of targeted therapies seen in clear-cell renal cell carcinoma (ccRCC) translate to RCC patients with non–clear-cell histology. There are several relevant non–clear-cell histologies including (in order of decreasing frequency) papillary, chromophobe, and collecting duct. Furthermore, any histology can be admixed with a sarcomatoid component, which is a particularly aggressive subtype.

Papillary Renal Cell Carcinoma

Papillary RCC (PRCC) is the most prevalent form of non-ccRCC and represents about 10%–15% of all cases of RCC. PRCC is subdivided into two distinct classes (type I and type II); clinically, type II disease is more aggressive. Antonelli et al. assessed a series of 132 patients with localized PRCC—57 patients (43%) had type I disease and 75 (57%) had type II disease.[1] Patients with type II disease had a significantly shorter disease-free survival (DFS). In a separate series of 130 patients with PRCC, 5 of 68 patients (7%) with type I disease died of cancer-specific causes compared with 27% with type II disease ($P = 0.002$).[2] In a series of 395 patients with PRCC, Fuhrman grade and tumor, nodal, and metastasis stages were independently associated with cancer-specific death, while PRCC subtype was not.[3] Other reports support the value of Fuhrman grade in predicting outcome in PRCC.[4,5]

Scant data are available to document outcomes of patients treated for metastatic PRCC prior to the era of targeted therapies. In a series of 38 patients with PRCC treated at a single institution between 1985 and 2005, median overall survival (OS) was 8 months.[6] The bulk of patients had received immunotherapeutic agents, and no responses were recorded. Responses to cytotoxic chemotherapy have also been dismal.

A Southwest Oncology Group protocol evaluated the efficacy of erlotinib in a series of 52 patients with PRCC. Among 45 evaluable patients, only 5 (11%) achieved a partial response (PR), but a median OS of 27 months was observed.[7]

Recently, efforts have been made to characterize the efficacy of vascular endothelial growth factor (VEGF)–directed therapies in PRCC. In a retrospective analysis, 53 patients were identified with papillary and chromophobe histology who had received sunitinib or sorafenib as initial treatment.[8] Of 41 patients with PRCC, median progression-free survival (PFS) of 7.6 months was observed, with a response rate (RR) of only 4.8%. Tannir et al. recently reported a phase 2 trial of sunitinib in 57 patients with non–clear-cell histology, including 27 patients (47%) with PRCC.[9] The median PFS for the entire cohort was 2.7 months and only 1.6 months with no objective responses for patients with PRCC.[9] Studies assessing VEGF–tyrosine kinase inhibitor (TKI) and pazopanib in PRCC and other non–clear-cell tumors are planned (Table 11.1).

Evidence exists for the benefit of mammalian target of rapamycin (mTOR) inhibition in PRCC. Approximately 20% of patients with advanced poor-risk RCC who were enrolled in the pivotal phase 3 trial comparing temsirolimus, interferon-alpha or the combination of the two possessed non–clear-cell histology.[10] Subset analyses from this study suggested that patients with non–clear-cell histology derived greater benefit from temsirolimus with respect to OS.[11] A phase 2 study of everolimus in non-ccRCC has recently been reported, with two objective responses (7%) among 29 patients with PRCC.[12] The median PFS in this series was 5.2 months. Recently, a great deal of attention has been focused on abrogation of MET signaling in PRCC. Several small-molecule MET inhibitors have been developed, with demonstrable preclinical activity in cell lines with both wild-type and mutated *MET*.[13] Foretinib (XL880/GSK089) demonstrated substantial affinity for MET as well as VEGFR (VEGF receptor), RON, AXL, and Tie-2.[14] A recently published phase 2 trial explored daily and intermittent dosing of foretinib in 74 patients with PRCC. A response rate of 13.5% was observed, with a median PFS of 9.3 months.[15] There are currently several other MET-directed therapies under evaluation in RCC.

Chromophobe Renal Cell Carcinoma

Chromophobe RCC is estimated to comprise about 5% of all cases of RCC.[16] The disease is characterized by an abundant eosinophilic cytoplasm, with an appearance akin to oncocytoma.[17] Chromophobe RCC can be distinguishable from oncocytoma, however, through the use of several immunohistochemical markers such as caveolin-1, MOC-31, CK7, S100A1, and claudin 8.[18,19] Gene rearrangements that may be specific to oncocytoma (eg, in the gene encoding cyclin D1, *CCDN1*) may also help distinguish these two entities. Chromophobe RCC is often thought of as a more indolent subset;

Table 11.1 Ongoing Trials for Patients With Metastatic Renal Cell Carcinoma With Non–Clear-Cell Disease

Trial Number	Number of Patients	Design	Description
NCT01524926	582	Phase 1: crizotinib	• Eligible tumor types: papillary mRCC (type 1) and other ALK/ MET-driven tumors (eg, sarcoma, anaplastic large-cell lymphoma) • No limit on prior therapy • Crizotinib: ALK inhibitor • 1° EP: RR
NCT01767636	39	Phase 2: pazopanib	• Eligible tumor types: non–clear-cell mRCC (including papillary, chromophobe, medullary, and sarcomatoid) • Up to one prior therapy • Pazopanib: VEGF–TKI • 1° EP: RR
NCT01108445	108	Randomized phase 2: sunitinib vs everolimus	• Eligible tumor types: non–clear-cell mRCC (excluding collecting duct, medullary, small cell, oncocytoma, or lymphoma-type) • No prior therapy • Sunitinib: VEGF–TKI • Everolimus: mTOR inhibitor • 1° EP: PFS at 6, 12, and 24 months
NCT01185366	108	Randomized phase 2: sunitinib vs everolimus	• Eligible tumor types: non–clear-cell mRCC (including papillary, chromophobe, collecting duct, sarcomatoid, translocation, and unclassified) • No prior therapy • Sunitinib: VEGF-TKI • Everolimus: mTOR inhibitor • 1° EP: PFS

1°, primary; ALK, anaplastic lymphoma kinase; EP, endpoint; mRCC, metastatic renal cell carcinoma; mTOR, mammalian target of rapamycin; PFS, progression-free survival; RR, response rate; VEGF–TKI, vascular endothelial growth factor–tyrosine kinase inhibitor.

10-year survival estimates for localized disease are in the range of 80% to 90%.[20,21] Furthermore, projections from the Surveillance, Epidemiology and End Results database suggest that chromophobe RCC accounts for only 1% of RCC-related deaths.[22] However, the existing literature does caution that there are several features of chromophobe tumors that may predict poor outcome, such as high grade, tumor necrosis, and sarcomatoid change.[23,24]

A predisposition to chromophobe RCC has been noted in association with Birt–Hogg–Dubé syndrome.[25] Defining the optimal systemic therapy for metastatic chromophobe RCC is challenging due to lack of data. In the previously cited series that included patients with non–clear-cell metastatic RCC (mRCC), 12 of 53 patients (23%) had chromophobe histology.[8] With first-line therapy including either sunitinib or sorafenib, three patients achieved a PR of 25%, with a median PFS of 10.6 months. The previously cited phase 2 trial by Tannir et al. that explored first-line sunitinib included only five patients with chromophobe histology.[9] With the caveat of this small sample size, an impressive median PFS of 12.7 months was reported, with two of the five patients achieving a partial response. The activity of mTOR inhibitors in chromophobe mRCC has not been adequately studied, although reports of response to these agents have been published.[22]

Sarcomatoid Renal Cell Carcinoma

Sarcomatoid elements can be present with any other subtype of RCC; these elements are marked by highly concentrated areas of spindle-like cells with substantial atypia.[26] Although historical series have estimated that approximately 5% of patients with RCC harbor sarcomatoid features, more recent series suggest the proportion may be as high as 10%–15%.[27–30] The presence of sarcomatoid elements is thought to portend a poor prognosis. The systemic management of sarcomatoid RCC can be dichotomized into two distinct approaches: therapy with cytotoxic chemotherapy and therapy with targeted agents. In a phase 2 trial of doxorubicin plus gemcitabine, 18 of 38 patients (47%) were noted to have pure sarcomatoid disease, while 13 patients (34%) had clear-cell disease with overlying sarcomatoid features.[31] One complete response and five PRs were observed, yielding an overall RR of 16%. An additional 10 patients had stable disease (SD) lasting at least 56 days. The median PFS was 3.5 months, and the median OS was 8.8 months. Given the dismal response to cytotoxic therapy alone, efforts have been made to evaluate the efficacy of targeted agents in sarcomatoid mRCC. Golshayan et al. reported outcomes from a series of 43 patients with mRCC and sarcomatoid features treated with VEGF-directed therapies (sunitinib, sorafenib, bevacizumab or sunitinib with bevacizumab).[32] Eight patients (19%) achieved a partial response, with an additional 21 patients (49%) achieving stable disease. Median PFS in this retrospective assessment was 5.3 months, with median OS of 11.3 months. In a series of 29 patients receiving temsirolimus or everolimus, 3 patients (10%) achieved a PR and 11 patients (10%) achieved SD.[33] Median PFS was 3.4 months, while median OS was 8.3 months.

To date, there are no prospective studies directly comparing cytotoxic and targeted therapies in sarcomatoid mRCC.

Xp11.2 Translocation Renal Cell Carcinoma

Translocations involving Xp11.2 were first associated with RCC more than two decades ago.[34–36] Although these aberrations were first noted in a pediatric population, the disease is recognized with increasing frequency in adults. The Xp11.2 translocation typically involves fusion of the transcription factor

E3 (*TFE3*) gene with either *PRCC* or the alveolar soft part sarcoma locus (*ASPL*).[37,38] These fusion products may have greater transcriptional activity and, in turn, promote carcinogenesis and tumor proliferation, given the role of TFE3 in mediating the cell cycle.[39]

Komai et al. assessed the frequency of Xp11.2 translocation in a series of 443 consecutively treated patients with RCC.[40] Although the overall incidence was low, 4 of 26 patients (15%) aged <45 years were noted to possess this aberration. Data related to outcomes with systemic therapy for metastatic Xp11 translocation RCC are sparse. Choueiri et al. assessed 15 patients who had received VEGF-directed therapies across a total of four institutions.[41] The majority of patients had metastatic disease at the time of initial presentation (8/15, 53%) and more than one metastatic site (12/15, 80%). These VEGF-directed therapies included sunitinib, sorafenib, and monoclonal anti-VEGF antibodies. Median PFS and OS were 7.1 months and 14.1 months, respectively. Although no prospective comparisons of targeted agents and immunotherapy are available, a report from the Juvenile RCC Network did document the activity of these agents retrospectively in a series of 23 patients with metastatic Xp11 translocation RCC.[42]

References

1. Antonelli A, Tardanico R, Balzarini P, et al. Cytogenetic features, clinical significance and prognostic impact of type 1 and type 2 papillary renal cell carcinoma. *Cancer Genet Cytogenet.* 2010;199(2):128–133.

2. Pignot G, Elie C, Conquy S, et al. Survival analysis of 130 patients with papillary renal cell carcinoma: prognostic utility of type 1 and type 2 subclassification. *Urology.* 2007;69(2):230–235.

3. Sukov WR, Lohse CM, Leibovich BC, Thompson RH, Cheville JC. Clinical and pathological features associated with prognosis in patients with papillary renal cell carcinoma. *J Urol.* 2012;187(1):54–59.

4. Klatte T, Anterasian C, Said JW, et al. Fuhrman grade provides higher prognostic accuracy than nucleolar grade for papillary renal cell carcinoma. *J Urol.* 2010;183(6):2143–2147.

5. Zucchi A, Novara G, Costantini E, et al. Prognostic factors in a large multi-institutional series of papillary renal cell carcinoma. *BJU Int.* 2012;109(8):1140–1146.

6. Ronnen EA, Kondagunta GV, Ishill N, et al. Treatment outcome for metastatic papillary renal cell carcinoma patients. *Cancer.* 2006;107(11):2617–2621.

7. Gordon MS, Hussey M, Nagle RB, et al. Phase II study of erlotinib in patients with locally advanced or metastatic papillary histology renal cell cancer: SWOG S0317. *J Clin Oncol.* 2009;27(34):5788–5793.

8. Choueiri TK, Plantade A, Elson P, et al. Efficacy of sunitinib and sorafenib in metastatic papillary and chromophobe renal cell carcinoma. *J Clin Oncol.* 2008;26(1):127–131.

9. Tannir NM, Plimack E, Ng C, et al. A phase 2 trial of sunitinib in patients with advanced non–clear cell renal cell carcinoma. *Eur Urol.* 2012;62(6):1013–1019.

10. Hudes G, Carducci M, Tomczak P, et al. Temsirolimus, interferon alfa, or both for advanced renal-cell carcinoma. *N Engl J Med.* 2007;356(22):2271–2281.

11. Dutcher JP, de Souza P, McDermott D, et al. Effect of temsirolimus versus interferon-alpha on outcome of patients with advanced renal cell carcinoma of different tumor histologies. *Med Oncol.* 2009;26(2):202–209.

12. Koh Y, Lim HY, Ahn JH, et al. Phase II trial of everolimus for the treatment of nonclear-cell renal cell carcinoma. *Ann Oncol.* 2013;24(4):1026–1031.

13. Bellon SF, Kaplan-Lefko P, Yang Y, et al. c-Met inhibitors with novel binding mode show activity against several hereditary papillary renal cell carcinoma-related mutations. *J Biol Chem.* 2008;283(5):2675–2683.

14. Qian F, Engst S, Yamaguchi K, et al. Inhibition of tumor cell growth, invasion, and metastasis by EXEL-2880 (XL880, GSK1363089), a novel inhibitor of HGF and VEGF receptor tyrosine kinases. *Cancer Res.* 2009;69(20):8009–8016.

15. Choueiri T, Vaishampayan U, Rosenberg JE, et al. Phase II and biomarker study of the dual MET/VEGFR2 inhibitor foretinib in patients with papillary renal cell carcinoma. *J Clin Oncol.* 2013;31(2):181–186.

16. Amin MB, Tamboli P, Javidan J, et al. Prognostic impact of histologic subtyping of adult renal epithelial neoplasms: an experience of 405 cases. *Am J Surg Pathol.* 2002;26(3):281–291.

17. Abrahams NA, MacLennan GT, Khoury JD, et al. Chromophobe renal cell carcinoma: a comparative study of histological, immunohistochemical and ultrastructural features using high throughput tissue microarray. *Histopathology.* 2004;45(6):593–602.

18. Kim SS, Choi YD, Jin XM, et al. Immunohistochemical stain for cytokeratin 7, S100A1 and claudin 8 is valuable in differential diagnosis of chromophobe renal cell carcinoma from renal oncocytoma. *Histopathology.* 2009;54(5):633–635.

19. Lee HW, Lee EH, Lee CH, Chang HK, Rha SH. Diagnostic utility of caveolin-1 and MOC-31 in distinguishing chromophobe renal cell carcinoma from renal oncocytoma. *Korean J Urol.* 2011;52(2):96–103.

20. Beck SD, Patel MI, Snyder ME, et al. Effect of papillary and chromophobe cell type on disease-free survival after nephrectomy for renal cell carcinoma. *Ann Surg Oncol.* 2004;11(1):71–77.

21. Przybycin CG, Cronin AM, Darvishian F, et al. Chromophobe renal cell carcinoma: a clinicopathologic study of 203 tumors in 200 patients with primary resection at a single institution. *Am J Surg Pathol.* 2011;35(7):962–970.

22. Shuch B, Vourganti S, Friend JC, Zehngebot LM, Linehan WM, Srinivasan R. Targeting the mTOR pathway in chromophobe kidney cancer. *J Cancer.* 2012;3:152–157.

23. Amin MB, Paner GP, Alvarado-Cabrero I, et al. Chromophobe renal cell carcinoma: histomorphologic characteristics and evaluation of conventional pathologic prognostic parameters in 145 cases. *Am J Surg Pathol.* 2008;32(12):1822–1834.

24. Paner GP, Amin MB, Alvarado-Cabrero I, et al. A novel tumor grading scheme for chromophobe renal cell carcinoma: prognostic utility and comparison with Fuhrman nuclear grade. *Am J Surg Pathol.* 2010;34(9):1233–1240.

25. Nickerson ML, Warren MB, Toro JR, et al. Mutations in a novel gene lead to kidney tumors, lung wall defects, and benign tumors of the hair follicle in patients with the Birt-Hogg-Dubé syndrome. *Cancer Cell.* 2002;2(2):157–164.

26. Shuch B, Bratslavsky G, Linehan WM, Srinivasan R. Sarcomatoid renal cell carcinoma: a comprehensive review of the biology and current treatment strategies. *Oncologist.* 2012;17(1):46–54.

27. Cheville JC, Lohse CM, Zincke H, et al. Sarcomatoid renal cell carcinoma: an examination of underlying histologic subtype and an analysis of associations with patient outcome. *Am J Surg Pathol.* 2004;28(4):435–441.

28. de Peralta-Venturina M, Moch H, Amin M, et al. Sarcomatoid differentiation in renal cell carcinoma: a study of 101 cases. *Am J Surg Pathol.* 2001;25(3):275–284.

29. Pal SK, Jones JO, Carmichael C, et al. Clinical outcome in patients receiving systemic therapy for metastatic sarcomatoid renal cell carcinoma: A retrospective analysis. *Urol Oncol.* 2013; 31(8):1826–1831.

30. Tandra P, Wang J, Loberiza FR, Hemstreet GP, Krishnamurthy J, Bhatt VR. Sarcomatoid renal cell carcinoma (SRCC): University of Nebraska Medical Center experience. *ASCO Meeting Abstracts.* 2013;31(6 Suppl):472.

31. Haas NB, Lin X, Manola J, et al. A phase II trial of doxorubicin and gemcitabine in renal cell carcinoma with sarcomatoid features: ECOG 8802. *Med Oncol.* 2012;29(2):761–767.

32. Golshayan AR, George S, Heng DY, et al. Metastatic sarcomatoid renal cell carcinoma treated with vascular endothelial growth factor-targeted therapy. *J Clin Oncol.* 2009;27(2):235–241.

33. Bastos DA, Voss MH, Karlo C, et al. mTOR inhibitor therapy for metastatic sarcomatoid clear cell renal cell carcinoma (ccRCC). *ASCO Meeting Abstracts.* 2013;31(6 Suppl):450.

34. Tomlinson GE, Nisen PD, Timmons CF, Schneider NR. Cytogenetics of a renal cell carcinoma in a 17-month-old child. Evidence for Xp11.2 as a recurring breakpoint. *Cancer Genet Cytogenet.* 1991;57(1):11–17.

35. Weterman MA, Wilbrink M, Janssen I, et al. Molecular cloning of the papillary renal cell carcinoma-associated translocation (X;1)(p11;q21) breakpoint. *Cytogenet Cell Genet.* 1996;75(1):2–6.

36. de Jong B, Oosterhuis JW, Idenburg VJ, Castedo SM, Dam A, Mensink HJ. Cytogenetics of 12 cases of renal adenocarcinoma. *Cancer Genet Cytogenet.* 1988;30(1):53–61.

37. Ramphal R, Pappo A, Zielenska M, Grant R, Ngan B-Y. Pediatric renal cell carcinoma: Clinical, pathologic, and molecular abnormalities associated with the members of the MiT transcription factor family. *Am J Clin Pathol.* 2006;126(3):349–364.

38. Argani P, Ladanyi M. Distinctive neoplasms characterised by specific chromosomal translocations comprise a significant proportion of paediatric renal cell carcinomas. *Pathology.* 2003;35(6):492–498.

39. Medendorp K, van Groningen JJ, Vreede L, et al. The renal cell carcinoma-associated oncogenic fusion protein PRCCTFE3 provokes p21 WAF1/CIP1-mediated cell cycle delay. *Exp Cell Res* 2009;315(14):2399–2409.

40. Komai Y, Fujiwara M, Fujii Y, et al. Adult Xp11 translocation renal cell carcinoma diagnosed by cytogenetics and immunohistochemistry. *Clin Cancer Res.* 2009;15(4):1170–1176.

41. Choueiri TK, Lim ZD, Hirsch MS, et al. Vascular endothelial growth factor-targeted therapy for the treatment of adult metastatic Xp11.2 translocation renal cell carcinoma. *Cancer.* 2010 116(22):5219–5225.

42. Malouf GG, Camparo P, Oudard S, et al. Targeted agents in metastatic Xp11 translocation/TFE3 gene fusion renal cell carcinoma (RCC): a report from the Juvenile RCC Network. *Ann Oncol.* 2010;21(9):1834–1838.

Chapter 12

Prognostic and Predictive Biomarkers in Renal Cell Carcinoma

David D. Chism and W. Kimryn Rathmell

The accelerated drug discoveries related to renal cell carcinoma (RCC), which are based on sizable gains in detailing relevant molecular biology, make the goal of personalized "tailored" therapy within reach. The application of biomarkers aids in this process by both assessing biological features that establish risk for metastases or disease recurrence (prognostic biomarkers) and/or by predicting which type of patient benefits from one of several targeted therapies or is more likely to encounter a specific side effect (predictive biomarkers). The standard tumor, nodal, and metastasis classification and conventional clinical prognostic factor models do not comprehensively address the rich complexities of a heterogeneous malignancy treated in the targeted-therapy era. In this chapter, we review the key prognostic and predictive biomarkers and discuss their evolving role in RCC.

Introduction

Prior to the current targeted-therapy era, individuals diagnosed with metastatic RCC (mRCC) had a median survival of 10 months and a 5-year survival rate of <10%.[1] The resistance of mRCC to conventional therapies ushered in a need for novel approaches. Since 2005, the US Food and Drug Administration (FDA) has approved seven RCC targeted therapies, which are divided into two major groups based on their molecular mechanism of inhibition: the mammalian target of rapamycin (mTOR) and the vascular endothelial growth factor (VEGF) pathway inhibitors.[2–9]

The pace of development of novel targeted therapies has created fertile ground for RCC biomarker discovery. As a result, a plethora of candidate prognostic and predictive biomarkers are in various phases of development and validation. Yet, none are FDA approved. In this chapter, we review the key validated prognostic biomarkers, including Fuhrman grade, sarcomatoid histological variant, nuclear protein Ki-67, and the insulin-like growth factor 2 (IGF-2) mRNA-binding proteins (IMP) 3. We evaluate the nonvalidated prognostic biomarkers categorized based on protein (carbonic anhydrase IX [CAIX], hypoxia-inducing factors [HIF] 1 and 2, and survivin), gene expression (clear cell type A [ccA] and B [ccB]), and cytogenetic abnormalities (chromosome 9p and 14q and BRCA1-associated protein-1 [BAP1]). We also discuss predictive biomarkers described based on predictions for activity of drugs targeting the mTOR or VEGF pathways.

Clinical Prognostic Factor Models

The University of California–Los Angeles integrated staging system is one of several clinical prognostic factor models (PFMs) used to assign nonmetastatic patients into groups in order to estimate risk for recurrence.[10–12] Unfavorable clinical PFMs for mRCC have also been well characterized. Motzer et al.[1] established a PFM that associated a poor survival in mRCC patients based on the following five criteria: Karnofsky performance status (<80%), serum lactate dehydrogenase (1.5 times the upper limit of normal [ULN]), hemoglobin (less than the lower limit of normal), serum calcium (>10 mg/dL), and absence of prior nephrectomy. Patients were divided into the following three groups: favorable (no risk factors; median survival 30 months), intermediate (one or two risk factors; median survival 14 months), and poor (three or more risk factors; median survival 6 months). This PFM was updated in 2002[13] with similar outcome data and prognostic criteria. Recent efforts to update these criteria for use in making prognostic assessments in the era of targeted therapies have identified many of the same features.[14] In addition, a neutrophil count greater than the ULN and platelets greater than the ULN were independent prognostic factors. These PFMs form the clinical framework on which tissue-based biomarkers will be interpreted, ultimately, in the form of integrated models.

Prognostic Biomarkers—Validated

Patients have the potential to benefit from prognostic biomarkers that are used to estimate risk of recurrent disease or other outcome. The validation process for generating biological markers for risk assessment consists of the following major phases: basic research for target identification, retrospective validation and development of an optimized test for clinical use, prospective clinical development, and FDA filing and approval. The majority of biomarkers currently being investigated are in the early basic research phase, resulting in an abundance of putative biomarkers, but only a handful that have been validated in independent retrospective series. A summary of the key validated biomarkers is provided here and in Table 12.1.

Fuhrman Grade

Nearly three decades ago, Fuhrman et al.[15] published a pivotal, landmark study in which the importance of nuclear histology in RCC prognosis was established. This qualitative assessment has since been widely incorporated into most clinical risk assessments as the single most widely reported criteria of tumor biology for clear cell RCC (ccRCC) tumors.

Table 12.1 Validated Prognostic Markers in Renal Cell Carcinoma

Biomarker	Type	Number of Patients	Results	Reference
Fuhrman grade	Retrospective	103	Grade 1 patients had no distant metastases at 5 years; grade ≥2 had 50% metastases at 5 years.	15
Sarcomatoid	Retrospective	108	Median OS, 17 months; regional or distant metastatic disease OS of 7.7 and 7 months, respectively: ($P < 0.004$)	16
Ki-67	Retrospective	224	High staining on tissue microarrays correlated with poor median survival (21 months; $P < 0.001$); combined with carbonic anhydrase IX, predicts survival based on low (101 months), intermediate (31 months), and high (9 months), respectively ($P < 0.001$)	17
	Retrospective	311	Presence of histologic necrosis correlated with higher Ki-67 staining ($P < 0.0001$) and had a lower 5-year disease-specific survival compared with patients without necrosis (36% vs 75%; $P < 0.0001$)	18
	Retrospective	741	High levels of Ki-67 more than doubled the risk of death from renal cell carcinoma (risk ratio, 2.18; $P < 0.001$); Ki-67 and coagulative tumor necrosis are not surrogates for each other in predicting poor outcome	19
IMP3	Retrospective	501	Localized tumors that did not express IMP3 had a longer metastasis-free survival and OS than those expressing IMP3 ($P < 0.0001$)	20
	Retrospective	716	Positive IMP3 expression was associated with a 42% increase in risk of death (hazards ratio, 1.42; $P = 0.024$)	21

IMP3, insulin-like growth factor 2 (IGF-2) mRNA-binding protein 3; OS, overall survival.

Sarcomatoid Variant

Sarcomatoid variant is an uncommon spindle-shaped histological variant that can be found in all subtypes of RCC and is also known for being a hallmark feature of an aggressive clinical course. To investigate its prognostic value, Mian et al.[16] performed a retrospective study of 108 patients with localized and advanced sarcomatoid RCC from 1987 to 1998 and established the poor outcomes associated with this feature ($P < 0.004$).

Nuclear Protein Ki-67

Nuclear protein Ki-67, an established marker of cancer proliferation, is also associated with more aggressive disease and poor prognosis if increased in RCC. Bui et al.[17] examined the tissue microarrays of 224 patients with ccRCC post-nephrectomy. Both Ki-67 and the expression of CAIX, a commonly expressed protein in ccRCC, were associated with clinical factors, pathology, and overall survival (OS). High Ki-67 staining correlated significantly with a poor median OS ($P < 0.001$), and low CAIX staining correlated significantly with poor median OS ($P < 0.011$). When combined for Ki-67 high expression and CAIX low expression, RCC tumors could be stratified into low-, intermediate-, and high-risk groups with median OS of 101, 31, and 9 months, respectively ($P < 0.001$). Similarly, Lam et al.[18] used both Ki-67 and CAIX to assess prognosis, and Tollefson et al.[19] implemented a subsequent validation study to confirm these findings in 741 tumor specimens from patients who underwent surgery for ccRCC. The prognostic information obtained for Ki-67 showed that high levels of Ki-67 more than doubled the risk of death from RCC ($P < 0.001$).

IMP3

IMP3 is a member of the IGF-II mRNA-binding protein family. It is absent in adult tissues, and its expression is found in developing epithelial tissue during human embryogenesis. Jiang et al.[20] investigated whether IMP3 could be used as a biomarker to predict metastasis and prognosis by examining 501 primary and mRCC tumors. They measured IMP3 mRNA and protein expression by quantitative real-time polymerase chain reaction and immunoblot, respectively. IMP3 expression was increased in both metastatic tumors and a subset of primary tumors. Localized tumors that did not express IMP3 had a longer metastasis-free survival and OS ($P < 0.0001$). This study suggests that IMP3 could be used in the early phases to identify patients with high potential to develop metastasis. Hoffman et al.[21] validated IMP3 as an independent prognostic marker for patients with ccRCC by studying 716 tumor specimens from patients. Expression of IMP3 was determined in 213 of the ccRCC specimens, with high expression associated with a 42% increase in the risk of death ($P = 0.024$); among patients with localized disease, it was associated with a 5-fold increase in the risk of distant metastases ($P < 0.001$).

Prognostic Markers—Nonvalidated

A summary of the nonvalidated prognostic biomarkers is provided here and in Table 12.2.

Table 12.2 Nonvalidated Prognostic Markers in Renal Cell Carcinoma

Biomarker	Type of Study	Number of Patients	Results	Reference
Protein				
CAIX	Retrospective	228	Of the 183 ccRCC tumors, patients with low expression had a less favorable prognosis than those with intermediate or high expression ($P = 0.012$ and $P = 0.001$, respectively)	22
			ccRCC CAIX is higher than in other subtypes	
	Retrospective	100	Poor prognosis in ccRCC patients without VHL mutation and low CAIX expression (median survival of 18 months)	23
HIF-2α	Basic research	In vitro,	Opposite of HIF-1α activity, HIF-2α enhances cell-cycle progression via c-Myc transcriptional activity in vitro; HIF-α subunit expression levels are responsible for cell-cycle progression	25
	Retrospective	160 tumors	ccRCC tumors could be classified as VHL wild type or VHL mutated and expressing both HIF-1α and HIF-2α (H1H2) or VHL mutated and expressing only HIF-2α	26
HIF-1α deletions	Basic research,	In vitro and in vivo,	Homozygous deletions of HIF-1α on chromosome 14q in ccRCC in vitro; downregulation of HIF-1α in HIF-1α cell lines promotes tumor growth; downregulation of wild-type HIF-1α promotes tumor growth in vivo	27
	Retrospective	52 tumors	Genetic and functional evidence for HIF-1α as ccRCC suppressor gene	

(Continued)

Table 12.2 (Continued)

Biomarker	Type of Study	Number of Patients	Results	Reference
Survivin	Retrospective	49	Significant correlation between survivin overexpression and high mortality rate (P < 0.05)	28
	Retrospective	75	Survivin expression was significantly higher than nontumor kidney tissues and absent in human kidney epithelial cell line	29
			Patients with high survivin levels had a significantly shorter OS than those with low levels (P < 0.001)	
			Survivin knockdown could enhance radiosensitivity and apoptosis	
RNA				
ccA, ccB outcome associated	Basic research, Retrospective	48 tumors	ccRCC is classified into two subclasses with different clinical outcomes; ccA had a markedly improved disease-specific survival compared with ccB (median survival of 8.6 vs 2.0 years; P = 0.002)	30
	Genomic, Retrospective	931 tumors	In a multivariate model, 16 genes remained significantly and strongly associated with recurrence-free interval after clinical/pathologic covariate and false discovery adjustments (HR, 0.68–0.80)	31
			Increased gene expression in angiogenesis-related (including EMCN and NOS3) and immune-related (including CCL5 and CXCL9) genes was associated with lower risk of recurrence	

DNA				
Chromosome 9p deletion	Retrospective	703	Deletions were found in 97 tumors (13.8%) and were larger and of high grade and high tumor classification and had lymph node or distant metastases ($P < 0.01$); median disease-specific survival in patients with localized disease who had deletions was 37 months compared with 82 months for those without deletion ($P < 0.01$)	32
Chromosome 14 q deletion	Retrospective	112	In nonmetastatic ccRCC, the loss of chromosome 14q was associated with higher stage (III or IV; $P < 0.001$), high risk for recurrence (2.78; $P < 0.002$), and decreased OS ($P < 0.03$)	33
			Gain of chromosome 8q was also associated with decreased survival	
Mutations	Whole genome, exome	7	Inactivated in 15% of ccRCC	34
BAP1 deletion			BAP1 deletion and PBRM1 regulate different gene expression, with BAP1 associated with higher tumor grade (q = 0.0005)	
BAP1 and PBRM1 mutations	Retrospective	145 + 327 (TCGA)	University of Texas Southwestern Medical Center tumors with BAP1 mutations had a worse median OS when compared with PBRM1 mutation (4.6 years vs 10.6 years; HR, 2.7; $P = 0.044$); TCGA tumors with BAP1 mutation also had a worse median OS when compared with PBRM1 (1.9 years vs 5.4 years; HR, 2.8; $P = 0.004$)	35

BAP, BRCA1-associated protein; ccRCC, clear cell renal cell carcinoma; ccA/B, clear cell carcinoma A/B; CAIX, carbonic anhydrase IX; HIF, hypoxia-inducible factor; HR, hazards ratio; OS, overall survival; TCGA = the cancer genome atlas; VHL, von Hippel-Lindau.

von Hippel–Lindau Gene and Carbonic Anhydrase IX

The von Hippel–Lindau (VHL) gene is the single most commonly mutated gene in ccRCC. The mutation, deletion, and hypermethylation of this gene are all inactivating events and have been examined with conflicting results for relation to outcomes. Thus, most attention to this high-frequency event in RCC development has been focused on downstream factors. CAIX is expressed in a majority of ccRCCs as a result of transcriptional activation by HIF-1α. Absent in normal renal tissue, it is overexpressed in ccRCC secondary to mutations in the VHL gene.[21]

Sandlund et al.[22] evaluated CAIX in ccRCC tumors from 228 patients based on low (0%–10%), intermediate (11%–90%), and high (91%–100%) expression. Patients with low expression had a less favorable prognosis than those with intermediate or high expression ($P = 0.012$ and $P = 0.001$, respectively). Not only did this study demonstrate increased expression of CAIX in ccRCC when compared with other subtypes (ie, papillary and chromophobe RCC), it showed less favorable prognosis with tumors that express low levels of CAIX. Patard et al also confirmed the correlation of lower protein expression of CAIX and poor prognosis.[23] CAIX expression was found to be an independent prognostic factor, with low CAIX expression associated with a poor clinicopathological phenotype and diminished survival.

Hypoxia-Inducing Factor–1α and –2α

HIF is a large heterodimeric transcription factor complex that consists of an unstable α subunit that binds with a stable β subunit in adaptation to hypoxia. HIF-1α has been well characterized for its role in angiogenesis, invasion, and metastasis. HIF-2α is a highly similar family member that transcriptionally activates a similar, but nonoverlapping, set of genes.[24]

The importance of HIF-2α in tumor promotion is being actively pursued with increasing clarity for its role in ccRCC. Gordan et al.[25] studied the differential effects of the HIF-α subunits in vitro and found that HIF-2α promoted c-myc transcriptional activity and cell-cycle progression in vitro, directly opposing the cell-cycle inhibitory activity of HIF-1α. Subsequently, this group demonstrated that ccRCC tumors could be classified as VHL wild type or VHL mutated and expressing both HIF-1α and HIF-2α (H1H2) or as VHL mutated and expressing only HIF-2α.[26] This cohort of tumors confirmed the predicted effect of HIF-2α on myc-dependent proliferation while also demonstrating a specific pattern of metabolic gene expression and activation of the mTOR pathway in H1H2 and VHL wild-type tumors. Additional clinical studies to measure both HIF-α subunit levels for patients with ccRCC in relation to either mTOR or VEGF-targeted therapy are ongoing.

Hypoxia-Inducing Factor–1α Deletion

HIF-α subunits have been clarified, with increasing importance placed on HIF-2α for cell-cycle progression in ccRCC. Shen et al.[27] introduced the new paradigm of HIF-1α acting in ccRCC as a tumor suppressor gene. Downregulation of HIF-1α promoted tumor cell growth of RCC4 cells in vivo, and gene expression found diminished evidence of the HIF-1α gene signature in tumors that sustained a 14q deletion spanning the HIF-1α locus

($P < 0.01$). Taken together, these data suggest that HIF-2α is the dominant tumor promoting transcription factor subunit of this family of proteins in ccRCC. However, even as tightly integrated as these proteins are with RCC tumorigenesis, their functional role in assigning prognosis is not known.

Survivin

Survivin, a key member of the inhibitors of apoptosis proteins, is upregulated in several malignancies.[28] Survivin (also BRIC5) plays a prominent role in the maintenance of cancer viability and chemoradioresistance. Lei et al.[29] assessed the prognostic significance of survivin expression in tissue samples from 75 patients. Expression of survivin mRNA was significantly higher in tumors than in nontumor kidney tissues. In addition, patients with high survivin levels had a significantly shorter OS ($P < 0.001$). This study supports the potential use of survivin as an independent, prognostic biomarker. Zamparese et al.[28] also investigated the use of survivin in ccRCC as a predictor of progression and survival. Using immunohistochemical techniques to assess survivin protein from 49 nonmetastatic ccRCC tumors, they found a significant correlation between survivin overexpression and mortality rate ($P < 0.05$). These data support survivin expression in ccRCC as a tool for identifying patients with more aggressive disease and a worse prognosis.

Gene Expression Signature Biomarkers

With modern gene expression methodologies, ccRCC can be further classified into two major subtypes based on inherent patterns of expressed genes. These biologically defined subgroups have been labeled clear cell A and clear cell B (ccA and ccB, respectively).[30] The two subtypes were validated in a second independent dataset ($N = 177$). The ccA subtype was associated with a significant improved survival relative to ccB subtype ($P = 0.0002$). Thus, like so many other tumor types, complex gene signatures can accurately stratify histologically similar tumors into groups that are both biologically and clinically meaningful. Other expression-based biomarker gene sets have been developed using a priori outcome case selections to identify signatures of genes associated with disease recurrence. These sets are also undergoing validation.[31]

Cytogenetics—Chromosomes 9p and 14q Deletions

Cytogenetic abnormalities play a crucial role in numerous malignancies. Chromosomal 9p deletion has been demonstrated to be associated with an aggressive phenotype of ccRCC. La Rochelle et al.[32] analyzed 703 ccRCC tumors using fluorescence in situ hybridization and cytogenetics. Ninety-seven tumors (13.8%) had deletions of chromosome 9p. When stratified for 9p deletion, they found that the 9p-deleted tumors were larger and had a high grade, a high tumor classification, and an increased lymph node or distant metastases ($P < 0.01$). Deletion of chromosome 14q is even more common in ccRCC than chromosome 9p deletions and is also associated with poor outcomes. Monzon et al.[33] examined tumor specimens from 112 ccRCC patients using 250K single-nucleotide polymorphism (SNP) microarrays. In nonmetastatic ccRCC, the loss of 14q was associated with higher grade

(III–IV; $P < 0.001$) and higher risk of recurrence (2.78; $P < 0.002$), as well as with decreased OS ($P < 0.03$). Intriguingly, they also determined that a gain of 8q conferred decreased OS ($P < 0.0001$). With HIF-1α residing on 14q, these findings corroborate data that implicate loss of this factor as a potential step in disease progression. The remaining genes implicated in these chromosomal regions remain to be determined.

BAP1 Mutation

Whole-genome and exome sequencing continues to push the discovery of important genetic contributors in ccRCC. Peña-Llopis et al.[34] used these techniques with tumor graft analyses to identify BAP1 as a putative two-hit tumor suppressor gene inactivated in 15% and associated with a higher tumor grade ($q = 0.0005$). BAP1 and PBRM1 anticorrelated in tumors ($P = 0.0005$), and when mutations of both were detected, these tumors were observed to have rhabdoid features characterized by an abundant acidophilic cytoplasm, acentric nuclei, and prominent macronucleoli, all characteristic of high-grade tumors. To determine the impact of these mutational events on clinical outcomes and to implicate BAP1 mutation as a potential prognostic biomarker, Kapur et al.[35] performed a retrospective analysis of two independent cohorts and showed that BAP1 mutations had a worse median OS when compared to PBRM1 mutation (4.6 years versus 10.6 years; hazard ratio [HR], 2.7; $P = 0.044$). This gene event, which remains to be prospectively validated, represents the first major genetic change with prognostic significance for ccRCC.

Predictive Biomarkers

RCC predictive biomarkers hold tremendous promise in weighing therapeutic options. A summary of the predictive biomarkers is provided here and in Table 12.3.

mTOR Pathway

Akt and Phosphorylated S6K (pS6)
Akt, also known as protein kinase B, is part of a pathway that links extracellular growth signals to mTOR activation, and its activity is marked by phosphorylation (pAkt). The S6 protein is phosphorylated by the pS6 kinase in the presence of active mTOR and is responsible for protein translation. Pantuck et al.[36] linked both Akt and pS6 with RCC. Levels of expression were correlated with OS. The relationship of these indicators of the greater mTOR pathway activation and response to mTOR inhibitor therapy remains an important category of putative biomarkers for prediction of response. However, these putative predictive biomarkers remain to be validated further for widespread use in making mTOR inhibitor therapy treatment decisions.

Lactate Dehydrogenase as a Predictive Biomarker of mTOR Outcome
High serum lactic acid dehydrogenase (LDH; 1.5 times ULN) is one of the five clinical factors used in Motzer's clinical prognostic model for mRCC.[1,13] Armstrong et al.[37] retrospectively investigated the role of LDH as a predictive biomarker in 404 poor-risk mRCC patients treated with the mTOR inhibitor

Table 12.3 Potential Predictive Markers in Renal Cell Carcinoma

Biomarker	Drug	Number of Patients	Results	Reference
mTOR-pathway–based therapy				
Akt/ pS6	Interleukin 2	375	By multivariate Cox regression analysis; tumor, nodal, and metastasis classification; Eastern Cooperative Oncology Group performance status; cytoplasmic and nuclear Akt, phosphatase and tensin homolog; and pS6 were independent prognostic factors of disease-specific survival	36
	Temsirolimus or interferon α	404	For poor-risk renal cell carcinoma, serum LDH is a predictive biomarker for the survival benefit with mammalian target of rapamycin inhibition	37
			Multivariable hazards ratio for death was 2.81 ($P < 0.001$) for patients with LDH >1 × ULN; of 140 patients with LDH above the ULN, overall survival was significantly improved with temsirolimus (6.9 months vs 4.2 months; $P < 0.002$)	
VEGF receptor pathway–based therapy				
Hypertension	Sunitinib	63	A combination of VEGF SNP 936 and VEGFR SNP 889 p was associated with overall survival ($P = 0.03$)	38
			VEGF SNP 634 was associated with the prevalence and duration of sunitinib-induced hypertension in univariable and multivariable analyses ($P = 0.03$ and $P = 0.01$, respectively)	
Cytokines and angiogenic factors	Pazopanib	215 (phase 2) 344 (phase 3)	High concentrations of interleukin 6 were predictive of improved relative progression-free survival benefit from pazopanib compared with placebo ($P_{interaction} = 0.009$)	39

LDH, lactic acid dehydrogenase; pS6, phosphorylated S6; SNP, single nucleotide polymorphism; ULN, upper limit of normal; VEGF, vascular endothelial growth factor; VEGFR, vascular endothelial growth factor receptor.

CHAPTER 12 **Biomarkers in Renal Cell Carcinoma**

temsirolimus. When compared with patients who had LDH less than or equal to normal, patients with an LDH that was greater than normal had an HR for death of 2.81 ($P < 0.001$). One-hundred and forty patients with an LDH greater than the ULN had a significant improvement in OS with temsirolimus (6.9 months versus 4.2 months; $P < 0.002$).

VEGF Pathway

VEGF and VEGFR SNPs and Hypertension

Hypertension is a well-documented on-target side effect of VEGF pathway inhibition. However, the extent of hypertensive response varies from patient to the patient, suggesting that there may be an element of host-specific interaction that may translate to tumor responses to therapy. Kim et al.[38] examined the association of VEGF and VEGFR2 SNPs with acquired hypertension and clinical outcome in metastatic ccRCC in patients treated with sunitinib. Sixty-three patients were treated with sunitinib; blood pressure data were monitored and germline DNA was retrospectively evaluated. Both VEGF and VEGFR2 SNPs were associated with the development of hypertension and further associated with response. A combination of VEGF SNP 936 and VEGFR SNP 889, when adjusted for prognostic group, was associated with OS ($P = 0.03$).

Interleukin 6 as a Predictor of VEGFR Tyrosine Kinase Inhibitor Outcome

Tran et al.[39] used a three-step approach—screening, confirmation, validation—to assess cytokine and angiogenic factors (CAFs) as prognostic and predictive biomarkers for patients treated with pazopanib. They screened the CAFs of 17 mRCC patients who had the greatest or least tumor shrinkage in a phase 2 trial; the result was the following five candidate markers: interleukin (IL)-6, IL-8, hepatocyte growth factor, tissue inhibitor of metalloproteinases, and E-selectin. Finally, in a randomized, phase 3 trial ($N = 344$ patients), they validated that high concentrations of IL-6 predicted improved relative progression-free survival benefit in patients treated with pazopanib when compared with placebo ($P_{interaction} = 0.009$). Validation of IL-6 as a predictive biomarker for treatment with mTOR inhibitors and other risk groups is also warranted.

Conclusions

Medical oncologists face significant challenges in determining which targeted therapy is best suited for their individual patient's tumor biology. Expanded treatment choices afforded by the RCC accelerated drug development program further complicate the evolving treatment landscape. Prognostic and predictive markers hold promise in fashioning personalized therapy. By molecularly staging mRCC patients based on KI-67 or IMP3 expression levels, physicians may determine prognosis and anticipated life expectancy, although more precise tools remain to be validated prospectively. Furthermore, continued headway into molecular biology and pathways coupled with growth in the field of genomics and proteomics will only hasten drug development, making the effective use of predictive RCC biomarkers markers crucial. Additional predictive biomarkers such as CAIX and members of the mTOR pathway are under investigation. As 7 RCC targeted therapies grow into 17 and as adjuvant therapies that can reduce risk for disease recurrence are developed, the patient will ask, Doctor, which therapy is right for me? Clinical and biological biomarkers are needed to provide coordinated information for providing a precise answer.

References

1. Motzer RJ, Mazumdar M, Bacik J, Berg W, Amsterdam A, Ferrara J. Survival and prognostic stratification of 670 patients with advanced renal cell carcinoma. *J Clin Oncol*. 1999;17: 2530–2540.

2. Hudes G, Carducci M, Tomczak P, et al. Temsirolimus, interferon alfa, or both for advanced renal-cell carcinoma. *N Engl J Med*. 2007;356: 2271–2281.

3. Motzer RJ, Escudier B, Oudard S, et al. Efficacy of everolimus in advanced renal cell carcinoma: a double-blind, randomised, placebo-controlled phase III trial. *Lancet*. 2008;372:449–456.

4. Escudier B, Eisen T, Stadler WM, et al. Sorafenib in advanced clear-cell renal-cell carcinoma. *N Engl J Med*. 2007;356:125–134.

5. Motzer RJ, Hutson TE, Tomczak P, et al. Sunitinib versus interferon alfa in metastatic renal-cell carcinoma. *N Engl J Med*. 2007;356:115–124.

6. Escudier B, Pluzanska A, Koralewski P, et al. Bevacizumab plus interferon alfa-2a for treatment of metastatic renal cell carcinoma: a randomised, double-blind phase III trial. *Lancet*. 2007;370:2103–2111.

7. Sternberg CN, Davis ID, Mardiak J, et al. Pazopanib in locally advanced or metastatic renal cell carcinoma: results of a randomized phase III trial. *J Clin Oncol*. 2010;28:1061–1068.

8. Rini BI, Escudier B, Tomczak P, et al. Comparative effectiveness of axitinib versus sorafenib in advanced renal cell carcinoma (AXIS): a randomised phase 3 trial. *Lancet*. 2011;378:1931–1939.

9. Motzer RJ, Hutson TE, Tomczak P, et al. Overall survival and updated results for sunitinib compared with interferon alfa in patients with metastatic renal cell carcinoma. *J Clin Oncol*. 2009;27:3584–3590.

10. Zisman A, Pantuck AJ, Wieder J, et al. Risk group assessment and clinical outcome algorithm to predict the natural history of patients with surgically resected renal cell carcinoma. *J Clin Oncol*. 2002;20:4559–4566.

11. Frank I, Blute ML, Cheville JC, Lohse CM, Weaver AL, Zincke H. An outcome prediction model for patients with clear cell renal cell carcinoma treated with radical nephrectomy based on tumor stage, size, grade and necrosis: the SSIGN score. *J Urol*. 2002;168:2395–2400.

12. Kattan MW, Reuter V, Motzer RJ, Katz J, Russo P. A postoperative prognostic nomogram for renal cell carcinoma. *J Urol*. 2001;166: 63–67.

13. Motzer RJ, Bacik J, Murphy BA, Russo P, Mazumdar M. Interferon-alfa as a comparative treatment for clinical trials of new therapies against advanced renal cell carcinoma. *J Clin Oncol*. 2002;20: 289–296.

14. Heng DY, Xie W, Regan MM, et al. Prognostic factors for overall survival in patients with metastatic renal cell carcinoma treated with vascular endothelial growth factor-targeted agents: results from a large, multicenter study. *J Clin Oncol*. 2009;27: 5794–5799.

15. Fuhrman SA, Lasky LC, Limas C. Prognostic significance of morphologic parameters in renal cell carcinoma. *Am J Surg Pathol*. 1982;6:655–663.

16. Mian BM, Bhadkamkar N, Slaton JW, et al. Prognostic factors and survival of patients with sarcomatoid renal cell carcinoma. *J Urol.* 2002;167:65–70.

17. Bui MH, Visapaa H, Seligson D, et al. Prognostic value of carbonic anhydrase IX and KI-67 as predictors of survival for renal clear cell carcinoma. *J Urol.* 2004;171:2461–2466.

18. Lam JS, Shvarts O, Said JW, et al. Clinicopathologic and molecular correlations of necrosis in the primary tumor of patients with renal cell carcinoma. *Cancer.* 2005;103:2517–2525.

19. Tollefson MK, Thompson RH, Sheinin Y, et al. Ki-67 and coagulative tumor necrosis are independent predictors of poor outcome for patients with clear cell renal cell carcinoma and not surrogates for each other. *Cancer.* 2007;110:783–790.

20. Jiang Z, Chu PG, Woda BA, et al. Analysis of RNA-binding protein IMP3 to predict metastasis and prognosis of renal-cell carcinoma: a retrospective study. *Lancet Oncol.* 2006;7:556–564.

21. Hoffmann NE, Sheinin Y, Lohse CM, et al. External validation of IMP3 expression as an independent prognostic marker for metastatic progression and death for patients with clear cell renal cell carcinoma. *Cancer.* 2008;112:1471–1479.

22. Sandlund J, Oosterwijk E, Grankvist K, Oosterwijk-Wakka J, Ljungberg B, Rasmuson T. Prognostic impact of carbonic anhydrase IX expression in human renal cell carcinoma. *BJU Int.* 2007;100:556–560.

23. Patard JJ, Fergelot P, Karakiewicz PI, et al. Low CAIX expression and absence of VHL gene mutation are associated with tumor aggressiveness and poor survival of clear cell renal cell carcinoma. *Int J Cancer.* 2008;123:395–400.

24. Hu CJ, Wang LY, Chodosh LA, Keith B, Simon MC. Differential roles of hypoxia-inducible factor 1α (HIF-1α) and HIF-2α in hypoxic gene regulation. *Mol Cell Biol.* 2003;23:9361–9374.

25. Gordan JD, Bertout JA, Hu CJ, Diehl JA, Simon MC. HIF-2alpha promotes hypoxic cell proliferation by enhancing c-myc transcriptional activity. *Cancer Cell.* 2007;11:335–347.

26. Gordan JD, Lal P, Dondeti VR, et al. HIF-alpha effects on c-myc distinguish two subtypes of sporadic VHL-deficient clear cell renal carcinoma. *Cancer Cell.* 2008;14:435–446.

27. Shen C, Beroukhim R, Schumacher SE, et al. Genetic and functional studies implicate HIF1α as a 14q kidney cancer suppressor gene. *Cancer Discov.* 2011;1(3):222–235.

28. Zamparese R, Pannone G, Santoro A, et al. Survivin expression in renal cell carcinoma. *Cancer Invest* 2008;26:929–935.

29. Lei Y, Geng Z, Guo-Jun W, He W, Jian-Lin Y. Prognostic significance of survivin expression in renal cell cancer and its correlation with radioresistance. *Mol Cell Biochem.* 2010;344:23–31.

30. Brannon AR, Reddy A, Seiler M, et al. Molecular Stratification of Clear Cell Renal Cell Carcinoma by Consensus Clustering Reveals Distinct Subtypes and Survival Patterns. *Genes Cancer.* 2010;1(2):152–163.

31. Rini BI, Zhou M, Aydin H, et al. Genetic and molecular predictors in genitourinary malignancies. *J Clin Oncol.* 2010;28:15s (suppl; abstr 4501).

32. La Rochelle J, Klatte T, Dastane A, et al. Chromosome 9p deletions identify an aggressive phenotype of clear cell renal cell carcinoma. *Cancer.* 2010;116(20):4696–4702.

33. Monzon FA, Alvarez K, Peterson L, et al. Chromosome 14q loss defines a molecular subtype of clear-cell renal cell carcinoma associated with poor prognosis. *Mod Pathol.* 2011;24(11):1470–1479.

34. Peña-Llopis S, Vega-Rubín-de-Celis S, Liao A, et al. BAP1 loss defines a new class of renal cell carcinoma. *Nat Genet.* 2012;44(7):751–759.

35. Kapur P, Peña-Llopis S, Christie A, et al. Effects on survival of BAP1 and PBRM1 mutations in sporadic clear-cell renal-cell carcinoma: a retrospective analysis with independent validation. *Lancet Oncol.* 2013;14(2):159–167.

36. Pantuck AJ, Seligson DB, Klatte T, et al. Prognostic relevance of the mTOR pathway in renal cell carcinoma: implications for molecular patient selection for targeted therapy. *Cancer.* 2007;109:2257–2267.

37. Armstrong AJ, George DJ, Halabi S. Serum lactate dehydrogenase predicts for overall survival benefit in patients with metastatic renal cell carcinoma treated with inhibition of mammalian target of rapamycin. *J Clin Oncology.* 2012;30(27):3402–3407.

38. Kim JJ, Vaziri SA, Rini BI, et al. Association of VEGF and VEGFR2 single nucleotide polymorphisms with hypertension and clinical outcome in metastatic clear cell renal cell carcinoma patients treated with sunitinib. *Cancer.* 2012;118(7):1946–1954.

39. Tran HT, Liu Y, Zurita AJ, et al. Prognostic or predictive plasma cytokines and angiogenic factors for patients treated with pazopanib for metastatic renal-cell cancer: a retrospective analysis of phase 2 and phase 3 trials. *Lancet Oncol.* 2012;8:827–837.

Chapter 13

Management of Complications of Targeted Therapies for Metastatic Renal Cell Carcinoma

Bradley Atkinson and Diana Cauley

Introduction

During the past decade, multiple targeted therapies received regulatory approval for metastatic renal cell carcinoma (mRCC). While greatly expanding the treatment armamentarium for mRCC, targeted therapies have a profile of adverse events (AEs) that is very different from that of traditional chemotherapy and immunotherapy.

Anti-Vascular Endothelial Growth Factor Monoclonal Antibody

Bevacizumab has been approved for use with interferon-alfa (IFN-α) for mRCC. The primary AEs seen in phase 3 clinical trials of bevacizumab and IFN-α therapy include fatigue, asthenia, hypertension, proteinuria, anorexia, and bleeding (Table 13.1). Additionally, toxicity of bevacizumab therapy includes gastrointestinal perforation (sometimes fatal), severe or fatal hemorrhage, and increased incidence of wound healing and surgical complications.[1,2]

Tyrosine Kinase Inhibitors

The oral tyrosine kinase inhibitors (TKIs) have a class AE profile characteristically unique, as compared with mammalian target of rapamycin (mTOR) inhibitors and conventional chemotherapy. Even among individual TKI therapies, the incidence and severity of AEs vary greatly, in part, based on their molecular targeted receptors, which include intended target and "off-target" toxicities and individual patient characteristics, such as comorbidities, tumor

Table 13.1 Incidence of Common Adverse Events of Targeted Therapies for Metastatic Renal Cell Carcinoma: >20%

System	Adverse Effect	Bevacizumab[1,2]	Everolimus[8]	Temsirolimus[7]	Sunitinib[14]	Sorafenib[15,16]	Pazopanib[16]	Axitinib[17]
Dermatologic	Hand–foot syndrome				+	+		+
	Rash		+	+		+		
	Alopecia					+		
	Hair color change						+	
Gastrointestinal	Nausea	+	+	+	+	+	+	+
	Stomatitis		+	+	+			
	Vomiting		+		+		+	+
	Anorexia	+	+	+		+	+	+
	Abdominal pain			+				
	Diarrhea	+		+	+	+	+	+
	Constipation			+		+		+
	Weight loss					+		+
	Mucosal inflammation				+			
Miscellaneous	Hypertension	+			+	+	+	+
	Asthenia	+	+	+		+		
	Fatigue	+	+		+			+
	Bleeding	+						
	Influenza-like illness	+						
	Pain			+				
	Headache	+						

	Dyspnea			+			+	
	Cough			+			+	
	Dysphonia							+
	Infection			+			+	
	Fever	+		+			+	
	Peripheral edema			+			+	
	Back pain			+			+	
Hematologic	Leukopenia				+	+		
	Neutropenia	+			+	+		
	Lymphopenia			+	+	+		+
	Thrombocytopenia				+	+		+
	Anemia			+	+	+		+
	Increased creatinine			+	+	+		+
Laboratory	Proteinuria	+		+				
	Hyperlipidemia		+					
	Increased lipase			+		+		+
	Increased aspartate aminotransferase			+	+	+		+
	Increased alanine aminotransferase			+	+	+		+
	Increased alkaline phosphatase			+				

(Continued)

Table 13.1 (Continued)

System	Adverse Effect	Bevacizumab[1,2]	Everolimus[8]	Temsirolimus[7]	Sunitinib[14]	Sorafenib[15,16]	Pazopanib[16]	Axitinib[17]
	Increased uric acid				+			
	Hypophosphatemia		+		+	+	+	
	Hypocalcemia					+	+	+
	Increased amylase				+			
	Hyperglycemia		+	+			+	
	Hypercholesterolemia		+	+				
	Hypertriglyceridemia		+					
	Total bilirubin increase						+	
	Hyponatremia						+	

extent and type, concomitant medications, and pharmacokinetics. Most AEs occur during early cycles of therapy and generally decrease in frequency with subsequent cycles.[3-5] Common TKI-associated AEs are listed in Table 13.1 and their prevention and management are reviewed in Table 13.2.

Mammalian Target of Rapamycin Inhibitors

Everolimus is an orally administered and temsirolimus is an intravenously administered inhibitor of mTOR kinase. Both medications have significant immunosuppressive properties and are associated with an increased risk of bacterial, fungal, and viral infections. Importantly, systemic fungal infections should be fully treated prior to starting therapy. Hepatitis B and C titers should be assessed prior to starting mTOR inhibitor therapy.[6]

mRCC treated with mTOR inhibitors can lead to elevation in serum creatinine, glucose, cholesterol, and triglycerides and to noninfectious pneumonitis (Table 13.1).[7,8]

Management Strategies of Selected Adverse Events

Rash

TKIs are associated with rash, more often with sorafenib, sunitinib, and axitinib (in descending order) than with pazopanib.[9] The rash associated with mTOR inhibitors is not as intense as that seen with TKIs and has a more maculopapular appearance. It may be associated with pruritis and often involves the face, scalp, and upper torso. For pruritic rash, antihistamines or anti-itch lotions may be indicated. For dry skin with or without pruritis, patients may use emollient-based moisturizers on a regular basis. Patients should also avoid exposing skin to hot water and sunlight so as to not worsen symptoms.[9]

Mucositis

Mucositis is characterized by painful inflammation and/or ulceration of the mucous membranes of the gastrointestinal tract; stomatitis refers to symptoms specifically in the mouth. Many patients experience pain, which can impact speaking, eating, or opening the mouth. Stomatitis is commonly seen in patients on sunitinib, sorafenib, bevacizumab/interferon alfa, temsirolimus, and everolimus. A number of management strategies are available, but there is no consensus regarding which one is most effective.[10] Mouthwashes that contain viscous lidocaine or those that are alcohol- and peroxide-free provide discomfort relief as well as help maintain good oral hygiene. If oral candidiasis is suspected, a nystatin suspension may be initiated.[9]

Diabetes Mellitus

Grade 3/4 hyperglycemia occurs in up to 15% of patients receiving mTOR inhibitor therapy. A management strategy for previously diagnosed diabetics is to frequently monitor blood sugar and adjust medications as necessary to

Table 13.2 Monitoring, Prevention, and Management Strategies of Common Adverse Events [10]

Adverse Event	Monitoring and Prevention	Management
Hand–foot skin reaction	• Pedicure before treatment in patients with plantar hyperkeratosis • Protect hands and feet and reduce exposure to hot water • Avoid constrictive clothing and excessive rubbing • Wear open shoes with padded soles • Avoid vigorous exercise or activities that place undue stress on the hands and feet; no excessive sport • Sorafenib: Oral vitamin B6 may prevent symptoms • Apply an alcohol-free moisturizer immediately after bathing; moisturizing cream can be applied sparingly on the hands and feet and can be worn at night under cotton gloves and socks • Patients at an increased risk of foot problems, for example, diabetes, need to pay careful attention to symptoms • Taking sunitinib in the evening may help to reduce the severity of hand–foot syndrome	• May include topical therapies for symptomatic relief; temporary treatment interruption, and/or dose modification; in severe or persistent cases, permanent treatment discontinuation may be required • Cooling foot or hand baths and shoe inlays may be used for relief of symptoms

Rash	• Sun exposure should be avoided
	• No intervention is required for grade 1 erythema and flushing
	• Intensified skin care and application of moisturizing lotion are useful
	• Management of dermatologic toxicities may include topical therapies for symptomatic relief, temporary treatment interruption, and/or dose modification; in severe or persistent cases, permanently discontinue
	• Gentle soaps, body washes, anti-dandruff shampoos, and corticosteroid shampoos may be used (fluocinonide 0.05%)
	• Treat rash with topical application of urea-containing lotion (5% urea ointment, methylprednisolone) or short-pulse oral corticosteroid therapy in refractory patients
	• Topical emollients, topical imidazole derivatives, and body lotions containing exfoliative alpha hydroxyl acid components may be used
	• Topical corticosteroids should be used judiciously; avoid long-term use of topical steroids (eg, betamethasone) because they increase the risk of topical infection
	• Seborrhoeic dermatitis-like rash on the face and scalp can be treated with antifungals (eg, ketoconazole 2% cream/ciclopirox 1% cream)
	• Antihistamines may be used
	• Patients with unusual lesions anywhere on the body should be examined by a dermatology consultant to rule out malignancy
	• In cases of skin erosion, the dose may need to be reduced or treatment stopped

(Continued)

Table 13.2 (Continued)

Adverse Event	Monitoring and Prevention	Management
Diarrhea	• Avoid foods that would aggravate the diarrhea • Favor food that can slow gastrointestinal motility, for example, bananas, rice, apples, toast • Avoid high-fiber foods, stool softeners, and fiber supplements	Dehydration management: • Aggressive oral rehydration with fluids containing water, salt, and sugar Pharmacological management: • Loperamide/diphenoxylate, standard dose (4 mg). followed by 2 mg every 4 hours or after every loose stool: more aggressive regimen: 4 mg, then 2 mg every 2 hours • Tincture of opium (0.6 mg in water every 3–4 hours), morphine, or codeine • Budesonide can be used to treat low- to medium-grade inflammatory bowel disease • Grade 3/4: interrupt treatment and/or reduce dose until symptoms subside to grade 1
Oral and gastrointestinal complaints	• Choose foods that do not require significant chewing • Avoid spicy/salty/acidic food and spirits; sweets are often well tolerated • Early intervention can help avoid dose reductions	Everolimus: • Use mouthwashes (without alcohol or peroxide) and topical treatments • Do not use antifungal agents unless fungal infection has been diagnosed • Perform endoscopy in severe cases • Dexpanthenol sugar-coated tablets, dexpanthenol cream, agents to protect the mucus membrane (Orabase, Gelclair, magic mouthwash), topical steroids, narcotic analgesics for pain relief (eg. lidocaine solutions, combinations of topical lidocaine) can be used • Mouth rinses (eg, sage tea, sodium chloride/baking soda solutions, with/without acetaminophen, and morphine or codeine) should be considered • For fungal infection, use oral nystatin, fluconazole, clotrimazole, amphotericin B, or pantoprazole; ketoconazole is contraindicated (may increase kinase inhibitor concentrations) • Antacids may be helpful

Fatigue/asthenia	• Monitor for anemia, hypothyroidism, cardiomyopathy, dehydration • Provide education and counseling • Encourage patients to conserve energy; reschedule activities to periods of peak energy; and stay active during the day to promote sleep • Stress management, relaxation techniques, and nutritional support may be helpful Dose adjustments: • Grade 3 or 4 fatigue requires treatment interruption or adjustment
Hypothyroidism	• Before starting sunitinib, measure thyroid function and treat any existing hypothyroidism • Observe patients on sunitinib closely for signs/symptoms of thyroid dysfunction
Hyperglycemia	• Optimize glycemic control in diabetic patients before initiating treatment with mTOR inhibitors • Adapt doses of or initiate insulin and/or hypoglycemic agent therapy • Advise patients to report excessive thirst or increase in volume or frequency of urination • Monitor fasting serum glucose before initiating treatment and periodically thereafter
Gastrointestinal perforation	• Monitor patients for early signs of gastrointestinal perforation, such as fever, abdominal pain, constipation, and vomiting • Discontinue treatment • Perform prompt surgical assessment
Hypertension	• Bevacizumab: monitor BP before and after each infusion (more frequently if BP is elevated) • Control hypertension before administration of bevacizumab or TKIs • Treat hypertension as needed with standard antihypertensive therapy (appropriate for the individual situation of the affected patient) • TKIs: monitor BP at least weekly during the first 12 weeks of therapy; frequency may be reduced thereafter if no BP elevations • If severe hypertension develops, suspend targeted therapy (and resume once hypertension is appropriately controlled) or permanently discontinue if medical control is not possible or hypertension becomes life threatening • For an individual patient, BP should be monitored using the same equipment throughout management

(Continued)

Table 13.2 (Continued)

Adverse Event	Monitoring and Prevention	Management
Cardiovascular events	• TKIs in patients with cardiac risk factors and/or history of coronary artery disease: obtain detailed cardiovascular history and perform physical examination for signs and symptoms of heart failure • Perform noninvasive evaluation of left ventricular function to detect subclinical cardiovascular disease • Primary focus should be ongoing, close monitoring for clinical signs and symptoms of heart failure • Exclude other etiologies of heart failure including hypothyroidism, anemia, and pulmonary embolism	Sunitinib: • In the presence of clinical manifestations of CHF, discontinuation of sunitinib is recommended; sunitinib should be interrupted and/or the dose reduced in patients without clinical evidence of CHF but with an ejection fraction <50% and >20% below baseline • Implement standard heart failure management
Hemorrhage	• Control hypertension • Avoid bevacizumab in patients with serious hemorrhage or recent hemoptysis • Use caution before initiating anticoagulant therapy in patients on bevacizumab • Patients receiving sorafenib and anticoagulants may be periodically monitored for complete blood counts (platelets), coagulation factors, and physical examination	• Patients receiving bevacizumab or TKIs should be educated about the management of minor bleeding such as epistaxis Bevacizumab and TKIs: • Any grade 3 or 4 hemorrhage should result in treatment discontinuation
Thromboembolism	• Thromboprophylaxis is recommended for hospitalized cancer patients (in the absence of bleeding or other contraindications)	• Prescribe low–molecular-weight heparins • Grade 3 VTE: interrupt dose, restart treatment if anticoagulation therapy is effective and patients do not present a risk of hemorrhage • Grade 4 VTE or arterial venous thromboembolism: discontinue treatment

Wound healing	• Bevacizumab should be discontinued at least 28 days before elective surgery and restarted after 28 days or when the wound is fully healed	• Monitor for incision-related complications
	• TKIs and mTORs should be interrupted (at least 1 week) before surgery and not reinitiated until adequate wound healing has occurred	• Assess for adequate wound healing
Pneumonitis	• Patients receiving temsirolimus or everolimus should be monitored for clinical respiratory symptoms	• Radiological changes only: monitor
	• Diagnosis should be based on pulmonary function tests, chest x-ray, and/or computed tomography scan; exclude opportunistic infection	• Radiological changes and moderate symptoms: consider temporary treatment interruption and/or dose reduction
		• Radiological changes and increasing clinical symptoms in conjunction with a decrease in diffusing capacity of the lung: drug discontinuation and corticosteroid treatment; treatment may be restarted at a lower dose on recovery to grade 1

BP, blood pressure; CHF, congestive heart failure; mTOR, mammalian target of rapamycin; TKI, tyrosine kinase inhibitor; VTE, venous thromboembolism.

prevent uncontrolled hyperglycemia. For nondiabetics, blood sugar should be screened frequently in order to monitor for new-onset diabetes. The oral biguanide, metformin, is a first-line choice for diabetes but is contraindicated if the creatinine clearance is <60 mL/min and must be held for 48 hours after radiologic scans.[9]

Hyperlipidemia

Grade 3/4 hyperlipidemia occurs in 3% of patients receiving mTOR inhibitors. Providers should draw an initial baseline lipid profile and again every 6 weeks if levels are elevated above recommended values.[9] The National Heart, Lung, and Blood Institute: Adult Treatment Panel III guidelines may be useful for managing patients with hypercholesterolemia and/or hypertriglyceridemia.

Hypertension

Hypertension in the general population is commonly treated according to the Joint National Committee on Prevention, Detection, Evaluation, and Treatment of High Blood Pressure (JNC7) guidelines. There are limited data regarding the management of hypertension in oncology patients. JNC7 guidelines may be followed; however, note that lifestyle modifications may be difficult for patients with decreased performance status related to their cancer diagnosis and treatment. Medications should be selected according to the patient's comorbidities, drug interactions, and compelling indications as well as contraindications. Traditional first-line medications include angiotensin converting enzyme inhibitors, angiotensin-receptor blockers, beta-blockers, calcium-channel blockers, and diuretics.[11] Providers may consider agents other than nifedipine, as it has been shown to induce vascular endothelial growth factor secretion. Providers should avoid the nondihydropyridine calcium-channel blockers, diltiazem and verapamil, for patients on TKI therapy due to CYP3A4 drug–drug interactions.[9]

Pneumonitis

Noninfectious pneumonitis is a class effect of the mTOR inhibitors; it is observed at higher frequency in patients receiving everolimus than temsirolimus.[12] Providers should perform careful clinical monitoring for this AE at each visit. Pretreatment pulmonary function tests may be needed, and chest computed tomography imaging should be performed if a patient presents with new respiratory symptoms. The optimal management of this AE is still undefined; however, in clinical practice, the use of corticosteroids is common. Albiges and colleagues have published a management guideline.[13]

Renal Issues

The incidence and severity of proteinuria are increased in patients receiving angiogenesis inhibitor therapy (ie, bevacizumab and the oral TKIs). In general, patients treated with angiogenesis inhibitors should have routine urinalysis monitoring. Patients with a urine dipstick reading ≥2 should have a 24-hour urine collection; therapy should be held for >2 grams of protein per 24 hours and resumed when proteinuria is <2 grams per 24 hours.[9]

A grade-1/2 rise in serum creatinine is common with bevacizumab and mTOR inhibitor therapy; treatment changes are not necessary. Rare grade-3/4 rises in serum creatinine warrant dose interruption and possible dose reduction.[6]

References

1. Escudier B, Pluzanska A, Koralewski P, et al. Bevacizumab plus interferon alfa-2a for treatment of metastatic renal cell carcinoma: a randomized, double-blind phase III trial. *Lancet*. 2007;370(9605):2103–2111.

2. Rini BI, Halabi S, Rosenberg JE, et al. Phase III trial of Bevacizumab plus interferon alfa versus interferon alfa monotherapy in patients with metastatic renal cell carcinoma: final results of CALGB 90206. *J Clin Oncol*. 2010;28(13):2137–2143.

3. Gore ME, Szczylik C, Porta C, et al. Safety and efficacy of sunitinib for metastatic renal-cell carcinoma: an expanded –access trial. *Lancet Oncol*. 2009;10(8):757–763.

4. Porta C, Szczylik C, Bracarda S, et al. Short- and long-term safety with sunitinib in an expanded access trial in metastatic renal cell carcinoma (mRCC). *J Clin Oncol*. 2008;26(s15):abstr 5114.

5. Sternberg CN, Hawkins RE, Szczylik C, et al. A randomized, double-blind phase III study (VEG105192) of pazopanib (paz) versus placebo (pbo) in patients with advanced/metastatic renal cell carcinoma (mRCC): updated safety results. *J Clin Oncol*. 2011;29(s7):abstr 313.

6. Di Lorenzo,G, Porta C, Bellmunt J, et al. Toxicities of targeted therapy and their management in kidney cancer. *Eur Urol*. 2011;59(4):526–540.

7. Hudes G, Carducci M, Tomczak P, et al. Temsirolimus, interferon-alfa, or both for advanced renal-cell carcinoma. *N Engl J Med*. 2007;356(22):2271–2281.

8. Motzer RJ, Escudier B, Oudard S, et al. Phase 3 trial of everolimus for metastatic renal cell carcinoma. *Cancer* 2010;116(18):4256–4265.

9. Appleby L, Marrissey S, Bellmunt J, Rosenberg J. Management of treatment-related toxicity with targeted therapies for renal cell carcinoma: evidence-based practice and best practices. *Hematol Oncol Clinc N Am*. 2011;25(4):893–915.

10. Eisen T, Sternberg CN, Robert C, et al. Targeted therapies for renal cell carcinoma: review of adverse event management strategies. *J Natl Cancer Inst* 2012;104(2):93–113.

11. Chobanian AV, Bakris GL, Black HR, et al. The Seventh Report of the Joint National Committee on prevention, detection, evaluation, and treatment of high blood pressure: the JNC 7 report. *JAMA*. 2003;289(19):2560–2572.

12. Atkinson BJ, Cauley DH, Ng C, et al. mTOR inhibitor associated noninfectious pneumonitis in patients with renal cell cancer: management, predictors, and outcomes. *BJU Int*. 2014;113(3):376–382.].

13. Albiges L, Chammings F, Duclos B, et al. Incidence and management of mTOR inhibitor-associated pneumonitis in patients with metastatic renal cell carcinoma. *Ann Oncol*. 2012;23(8):1943–1953.

14. Motzer RJ, Hutson TE, Tomczak P, et al. Sunitinib versus interferon alfa in metastatic renal-cell carcinoma. *N Engl J Med*. 2007;356(2):115–124.

15. Escudier B, Eisen T, Stadler WM, et al. Sorafenib in advanced clear-cell renal-cell carcinoma. *N Engl J Med*. 2007;356(2):125–134.

16. Sternberg CN, Davis ID, Mardiak J, et al. Pazopanib in locally advanced or metastatic renal cell carcinoma: results of a randomized phase III trial. *J Clin Oncol.* 2010;28(6):1061–1068.

17. Rini BI, Escudier B, Tomczak P, et al. Comparative effectiveness of axitinib versus sorafenib in advanced renal cell carcinoma (AXIS): a randomised phase 3 trial. *Lancet.* 2011;378(9807):1931–1939.

Chapter 14

The Role of Traditional and Stereotactic Radiation in Metastatic Renal Cell Carcinoma

Amol J. Ghia and Seungtaek Choi

Introduction

Renal cell carcinoma (RCC) is the seventh leading cause of death from cancer in the United States.[1,2] Bone is a common site of metastatic involvement, with 20%–35% of RCC patients eventually developing bone metastases.[3–5] In one series, more than one-third of patients with cancer had vertebral metastases on autopsy.[6] Spine metastases are not only the most prevalent skeletal metastases, they are also the cause of the most morbidity. Due to the weight-bearing function of the spine, vertebral compression fractures (VCFs) can occur when the vertebral bodies are compromised by metastases. While some spinal metastases are asymptomatic, the development of acute VCFs results in significant morbidity including pain, kyphosis, decreased mobility, neurologic complications, and, ultimately, a decline in performance status. Additionally, disease progression can lead to neurological deterioration due to compression of the spinal cord or cauda equina, which can lead to permanent disability if not addressed rapidly.[7] With improved progression-free survival (PFS) and overall survival (OS) rates owing to the use of targeted therapies in patients with metastatic RCC, addressing bone metastases with modalities that can provide durable local control has become a growing concern.[8,9] The majority of RCC patients with bone metastases will undergo some form of radiation therapy to palliate pain, prevent disease progression and pathological fracture, and halt or reverse neurological compromise.[10]

Conventional Radiotherapy

The mainstay of palliative treatment for RCC bone metastases has been conventional, fractionated radiation. Conventional radiotherapy is defined as radiation usually delivered using one or two beams without highly conformal techniques to the site of disease. As a result, critical structures such as bowel and spinal cord receive the full radiation dose. Typically, the total dose given is limited to doses below the tolerance level of the normal tissues; the daily dose given in 2.0- to 3.0-Gy fractions. This significantly limits the effectiveness of this technique, as doses below the normal tissue tolerance level may be significantly below the optimal therapeutic dose.[11–13] However, this technique has the advantage that it can be delivered quickly and can address multiple sites simultaneously. Though, for radioresistant tumors including RCC, conventionally fractionated radiation has been shown to lead to suboptimal local control.[14–16]

The role of hypofractionation has been addressed using this conventional technique. Several studies have addressed the role of palliative radiation delivered in a single fraction (typically 8 Gy), as compared with fractionated radiation. This question was studied in the context of a Radiation Therapy Oncology Group phase 3 clinical trial that randomized patients with bone metastases to either 8 Gy in a single fraction or 30 Gy in 10 fractions. Both regimens were equivalent with respect to pain control at 3 months, though the 8-Gy arm had a higher rate of re-treatment. While this study did not address metastatic disease in the spine specifically, patients with spinal metastases were included.[17] Dose escalation using these conventional beam arrangements was not possible due to potential toxicity to spinal cord and other critical structures.

Stereotactic Spinal Radiosurgery

Stereotactic spinal radiosurgery (SSRS) is a form of stereotactic body radiotherapy (SBRT) by which advanced treatment delivery techniques (eg, intensity-modulated radiotherapy) are combined with image guidance and rigid immobilization to deliver a high dose of conformal radiation to the target while minimizing dose to nearby critical structures such as the spinal cord. This is in contrast to conventional radiotherapy, which uses less conformal techniques and often without image guidance. Given the nonconformity of conventional treatment, the ability to deliver high doses of radiation is severely limited by the dose tolerance of the spinal cord. Patients who have spine metastases from radioresistant tumors such as RCC have poorer response to radiation treatment, shorter duration of response, and poorer survival, as compared with those with more responsive tumors (eg, breast cancer).[18]

In the 1990s, investigators started applying the stereotactic principles used in treating intracranial metastases to treating spinal metastases. Rigid immobilization is a hallmark of stereotactic radiosurgical techniques, and, historically, treatment of intracranial metastases used a head frame that was fixed to the patient's skull with pins. For SSRS, image-guided, noninvasive methods were developed.[13,19] Using rigid immobilization in the form of vacuum-locked bags and image guidance, treatment delivery accuracy is on the order of 1 mm.[13,20]

In a report by Gerszten et al., 115 patients received SSRS to 123 lesions with a median follow-up of 18 months. Of those presenting with pain, 74 of 79 (94%) patients experienced a reduction in pain after treatment.[21] In another report of 31 patients, rapid and significant pain relief was achieved after SSRS in 32 of 34 treated tumors.[22] In a phase 1/2 prospective report from the MD Anderson Cancer Center (MDACC), 63 patients underwent SSRS for spinal metastases. The actuarial 1-year tumor progression-free incidence was 84%. No late grade 3 or 4 toxicities were noted, with a median follow-up of 21.3 months. Complete pain relief was noted in 54% of patients at 6 months following SSRS treatment.[23] This compares favorably with conventional radiotherapy for bone metastases, which provides 0%–20% complete pain relief with the use of the brief pain inventory.[17,24]

A summary of the literature on the use of SSRS to treat RCC spine metastases is presented in Table 14.1. No grade 3 or grade 4 toxicities were noted in these studies. Gerszten et al. published a retrospective report on 48 patients with 60 RCC metastases to the spine treated with single-fraction SSRS and followed for a median of 37 months.[25] Pain improved in 34 of 38 patients (89%) who presented with pain, and radiographic control was noted in 7 of 8 patients treated primarily for radiographic progression. Nguyen et al. performed a retrospective study of 48 patients with 55 spinal metastases from RCC treated with SSRS.[26] The median follow-up was 13.1 months. The actuarial 1-year spine tumor PFS was 82.1%. Balagamwala et al. published a retrospective study of treated spinal metastases from RCC with SSRS.[27] Fifty-seven patients with 88 metastases were evaluated. The proportion of patients presenting with pain and achieving a complete pain response increased from 15.4% at 2 weeks post-SSRS to 66.7% by 9 months post-SSRS.

SSRS can also be used in patients who previously received conventional radiotherapy with subsequent progression. For these patients, repeat conventional radiation carries a significant risk for toxicity. Sahgal et al. reported on 37 patients previously irradiated who underwent subsequent SSRS for salvage.[28] Median OS was 21 months. The 1-year progression-free probability in tumors previously irradiated was 96%. Again, no radiation-induced myelopathy or radiculopathy was noted. Mahadevan et al. published their institutional experience in treating 60 patients in the re-irradiation setting.[29] With median OS of 11 months and PFS of 9 months, only 7% of patients showed disease progression at the treated site following SSRS. Garg et al. performed a prospective trial enrolling 59 patients with 63 tumors of the spine re-irradiated with SSRS.[30] With a mean follow-up of 17.6 months, the actuarial 1-year local control rate was 76% and the freedom from neurologic progression was 92%. Thirteen of the 16 tumors that progressed were within 5 mm of the spinal cord and were likely due to underdosing. Two patients had grade 3 neurologic toxicity. There was no grade 4 toxicity.

Another indication for SSRS is in the post-operative setting. Local recurrence following surgery with or without adjuvant radiation is common in long-term survivors, with actuarial rates as high as 58% at 6 months, 69% at 1 year, and 94% at 4 years.[31] In the post-operative patient, SSRS may be used to sterilize the operative bed.[32] Dedicated publications on the post-operative use of SSRS are sparse, but several retrospective reports are available. Crude local control rates range from 81% to 94%;[33–35] in one study, pain was improved in 24 of the 26 patients.[34] In a recent report from the Memorial Sloan Kettering Cancer Center, 186 patients with epidural cord compression

Table 14.1 Stereotactic Spinal Radiosurgery and Renal Cell Carcinoma

	Gerszten et al. University of Pittsburgh	Nguyen et al. MD Anderson Cancer Center	Balagamwala et al. Cleveland Clinic
Patients	48	48	57
Lesions	60	55	88
Median follow-up (months)	37	13.1	5.4
Dose/fx	14–20 Gy (median 16 Gy) in 1 fraction	30 Gy/5 fx (n = 13); 27 Gy/3 fx (n = 34); 24 Gy/1 fx (n = 8)	8–16 Gy (median 15 Gy) in 1 fx
Previous RT	42 of 60 lesions	26 of 48 patients	18 of 57 patients
Radiographic local control	7/8 (88%)	82.1% (actuarial 1 year)	71.2% (actuarial 1 year)
Pain response	34/38 (89%) improvement	64% pain free at 9 months	73.3% pain free at 9 months
Median overall survival	NR	22 months	8.3 months

underwent surgery followed by SSRS.[36] In those receiving high-dose SSRS, local failure rates were less than 10% at 1 year.

SSRS may be delivered using a variety of treatment machines and treatment algorithms based on the treating institution. Various immobilization devices, image-guidance techniques, and treatment delivery techniques may be used. At MDACC, patients typically receive one to three fractions of treatment with a dose between 18 Gy and 27 Gy to the gross disease and between 16 Gy and 21 Gy to areas at risk (eg, contiguous bone marrow).[37,38] The patient is immobilized in a BodyFix bag (by Elekta, Stockholm, Sweden) with a vacuum-sealed plastic covering for lower thoracic, lumbar, and sacral lesions. A large thermoplastic mask is sometimes used for cervical and upper thoracic lesions. Linac-based intensity-modulated radiotherapy techniques are used. On the day of treatment, the patient is positioned in the immobilization device; positioning is verified using kV dual X-rays (Exactrac by BrainLab, Feldkirchen, Germany; Westchester, Illinois, USA). Positioning is further verified using a cone beam computed tomography scan. A final check with port films and a second set of Exactrac images is then performed prior to treatment. Typically, nine treatment fields are used and positioning is reverified prior to each treatment field with Exactrac imaging.

Dose constraints on the spinal cord take precedence when performing dosimetric planning. As such, radiation myelopathy is a rare entity, and dose constraints that correspond to a 1%–5% risk of spinal cord toxicity have been published.[39] Although late neurotoxicity is exceedingly rare with SSRS, VCF has been noted to occur in 10%–39% of patients who receive SSRS.[40–42] Risk factors for VCF include age >55 years, a preexisting fracture, osteolytic process, baseline pain, and high dose per fraction.[40,42,43] One mechanism proposed for VCF is osteoradionecrosis, where healthy vertebral bone and tumor tissue are replaced by weak friable necrotic tissue.[41] Management of VCF ranges from percutaneous cement augmentation to open spinal reconstructive surgery, depending on individual clinical circumstances.

Stereotactic Body Radiotherapy

Stereotactic radiosurgery has also been used in the treatment of bone metastases outside of the spine and soft tissue metastases (eg, lung, liver). As with SSRS, SBRT requires patient immobilization and image guidance to deliver conformal doses of radiation to the target. The treatment is often given using a linear accelerator, although more specialized machines for stereotactic radiosurgery can be used (eg, the Cyberknife by Accuray, Sunnyvale, CA, USA).

Doses that have been used vary widely, ranging from 45 Gy × 10 treatments to 20 Gy × 3 treatments. Several studies that looked at the use of SBRT in RCC are summarized in Table 14.2. As can be seen, all of these studies have shown high local control at the site of metastatic disease, with very few side effects. However, additional studies are required to determine which patients will benefit the most from such treatments.

Table 14.2 Stereotactic Body Radiotherapy and Renal Cell Carcinoma

	Ranck et al.	Zelefsky et al.	Rusthaven et al.
Patients	18		38
Lesions	39	105	63
Sites of treatment	Bone (11) Lung (7) Liver (2) (RCC in 100%)	Bone (104) Lymph node (1) (RCC in 100%)	Lung (63) (RCC in 18.4%)
Dose/fx	24–48 Gy/3 fx or 42–50 Gy/10-14 fx	18–24 Gy/1 fx or 20–30 Gy/3–5 fx	4860 Gy/3 fx
Radiographic local control	91.4% at 2 years	44% at 3 years (88% for 24 Gy/1 fx)	96% at 2 years
Overall survival	85% at 2 years		39% at 2 years
Toxicity	15.3% grade 2 0% grade 3 or higher	5.7% grade 2 (2 for dermatitis, 4 rib fracture) 1.0% grade 4 (dermatitis)	7.9% grade 3 0% grade or higher

RCC, renal cell carcinoma.

Conclusions

Radiation therapy plays a major role in the treatment of bone metastases in patients with RCC. Although conventional radiation therapy remains the mainstay of treatment, stereotactic radiosurgery is playing an ever-increasing role in the palliative treatment of these patients due to an increasing body of literature that shows both increased efficacy and safety. However, radiosurgery does require additional professional and technical expertise compared with conventional radiation therapy; extra care should be taken when patients are considered for treatment with radiosurgery.

References

1. Adiga GU, Dutcher JP, Larkin M, Garl S, Koo J. Characterization of bone metastases in patients with renal cell cancer. *BJU Int.* 2004;93:1237–1240.

2. Pantuck AJ, Zisman A, Belldegrun AS. The changing natural history of renal cell carcinoma. *J Urol.* 2001;166:1611–1623.

3. National Cancer Institute. SEER Statistical Fact Sheets. http://seer.cancer.gov/statfacts/index.html. Accessed 8/27/2013.

4. Brown JE, Coleman.E. Metastatic Bone Disease: Developing Strategies to Optimize Management. *Am J Cancer.* 2003:2269–2281.

5. Woodward E, et al. Skeletal complications and survival in renal cancer patients with bone metastases. *Bone.* 2011;48:160–166.

6. Bhatt AD, Schuler JC, Boakye M, Woo SY. Current and emerging concepts in non-invasive and minimally invasive management of spine metastasis. *Cancer Treat Rev.* 2013;39:142–152.

7. Lo SS, et al. ACR Appropriateness Criteria (R) spinal bone metastases. *J Palliat Med.* 2013;16:9–19.

8. Flanigan RC, Campbell SC, Clark JI, Picken MM. Metastatic renal cell carcinoma. *Curr Treat Options Oncol.* 2003;4:385–390.

9. Coppin C, Kollmannsberger C, Le L, Porzsolt F, Wilt TJ. Targeted therapy for advanced renal cell cancer (RCC): a Cochrane systematic review of published randomised trials. *BJU Int.* 2011;108:1556–1563.

10. Gerszten PC, Mendel E, Yamada Y. Radiotherapy and radiosurgery for metastatic spine disease: what are the options, indications, and outcomes? *Spine.* 2009;34:S78–92.

11. Faul CM, Flickinger JC. The use of radiation in the management of spinal metastases. *J Neurooncol.* 1995;23:149–161.

12. Loblaw DA, Mitera G, Ford M, Laperriere NJ. A 2011 updated systematic review and clinical practice guideline for the management of malignant extradural spinal cord compression. *Int J Radat Oncol Biol Phys.* 2012;84:312–317.

13. Ryu SI, et al. Image-guided hypo-fractionated stereotactic radiosurgery to spinal lesions. *Neurosurgery.* 2001;49:838–846.

14. Onufrey V, Mohiuddin M. Radiation therapy in the treatment of metastatic renal cell carcinoma. *Int J Radat Oncol Biol Phys.* 1985;11:2007–2009.

15. Maor MH, Frias AE, Oswald MJ. Palliative radiotherapy for brain metastases in renal carcinoma. *Cancer.* 1988;62:1912–1917.

16. Wronski M, Maor MH, Davis BJ, Sawaya R, Levin VA. External radiation of brain metastases from renal carcinoma: a retrospective study of 119 patients from the M. D. Anderson Cancer Center. *Int J Radat Oncol Biol Phys.* 1997;37:753–759.

17. Hartsell WF. et al. Randomized trial of short- versus long-course radiotherapy for palliation of painful bone metastases. *J Natl Cancer Inst.* 2005;97:798–804.

18. Maranzano E, Latini, P. Effectiveness of radiation therapy without surgery in metastatic spinal cord compression: final results from a prospective trial. *Int J Radat Oncol Biol Phys.* 1995;32:959–967.

19. Murphy MJ, et al. Image-guided radiosurgery in the treatment of spinal metastases. *Neurosurg Focus.* 2001;11:e6.

20. Ryu S. et al. Image-guided and intensity-modulated radiosurgery for patients with spinal metastasis. *Cancer.* 2003;97:2013–2018.

21. Gerszten PC, et al. CyberKnife frameless stereotactic radiosurgery for spinal lesions: clinical experience in 125 cases. *Neurosurgery.* 2004;55:89–98; discussion 98–89.

22. Benzil DL, Saboori M, Mogilner AY, Rocchio R, Moorthy CR. Safety and efficacy of stereotactic radiosurgery for tumors of the spine. *J Neurosurg.* 2004;101(suppl 3):413–418.

23. Wang XS, et al. Stereotactic body radiation therapy for management of spinal metastases in patients without spinal cord compression: a phase 1-2 trial. *Lancet Oncol.* 2012;13:395–402.

24. Foro Arnalot P. et al. Randomized clinical trial with two palliative radiotherapy regimens in painful bone metastases: 30 Gy in 10 fractions compared with 8 Gy in single fraction. *Radiother Oncol.* 2008;89:150–155.

25. Gerszten PC, et al. Stereotactic radiosurgery for spinal metastases from renal cell carcinoma. *J Neurosurg Spine.* 2005;3:288–295.

26. Nguyen QN. et al. Management of spinal metastases from renal cell carcinoma using stereotactic body radiotherapy. *Int J Radat Oncol Biol Phys.* 2010; 76:1185–1192.

27. Balagamwala EH, et al. Single-fraction stereotactic body radiotherapy for spinal metastases from renal cell carcinoma. *J Neurosurg Spine*. 2012;17:556–564.

28. Sahgal A, et al. Stereotactic body radiotherapy is effective salvage therapy for patients with prior radiation of spinal metastases. *Int J Radat Oncol Biol Phys*. 2009;74:723–731.

29. Mahadevan A. et al. Stereotactic body radiotherapy reirradiation for recurrent epidural spinal metastases. *Int J Radat Oncol Biol Phys*. 2011;81:1500–1505.

30. Garg AK, et al. Prospective evaluation of spinal reirradiation by using stereotactic body radiation therapy: The University of Texas MD Anderson Cancer Center experience. *Cancer*. 2011;117:3509–3516.

31. Klekamp J, Samii H. Surgical results for spinal metastases. *Acta Neurochir*. 1998;140:957–967.

32. Sahgal A, et al. Stereotactic body radiotherapy for spinal metastases: current status, with a focus on its application in the postoperative patient. *J Neurosurg Spine*. 2011;14:151–166.

33. Rock JP, et al. Postoperative radiosurgery for malignant spinal tumors. *Neurosurgery*. 2006;58:891–898; discussion 891–898.

34. Gerszten PC, et al. Combination kyphoplasty and spinal radiosurgery: a new treatment paradigm for pathological fractures. *J Neurosurg Spine*. 2005;3:296–301.

35. Moulding HD. et al. Local disease control after decompressive surgery and adjuvant high-dose single-fraction radiosurgery for spine metastases. *J Neurosurg Spine*. 2010;13:87–93.

36. Laufer I. et al. Local disease control for spinal metastases following "separation surgery" and adjuvant hypofractionated or high-dose single-fraction stereotactic radiosurgery: outcome analysis in 186 patients. *J Neurosurg Spine*. 2013;18:207–214.

37. Garg AK. et al. Phase 1/2 trial of single-session stereotactic body radiotherapy for previously unirradiated spinal metastases. *Cancer*. 2012;118:5069–5077.

38. Weksberg DC. et al. Generalizable class solutions for treatment planning of spinal stereotactic body radiation therapy. *Int J Radat Oncol Biol Phys*. 2012;84:847–853.

39. Sahgal A. et al. Probabilities of radiation myelopathy specific to stereotactic body radiation therapy to guide safe practice. *Int J Radat Oncol Biol Phys*. 2013;85:341–347.

40. Boehling NS, et al. Vertebral compression fracture risk after stereotactic body radiotherapy for spinal metastases. *J Neurosurg Spine*. 2012;16:379–386.

41. Sahgal A, Whyne CM, Ma L, Larson DA, Fehlings MG. Vertebral compression fracture after stereotactic body radiotherapy for spinal metastases. *Lancet oncol*. 2013;14:e310–320.

42. Rose,PS. et al. Risk of fracture after single fraction image-guided intensity-modulated radiation therapy to spinal metastases. *J Clin Oncol*. 2009;27:5075–5079.

43. Cunha MV. et al. Vertebral compression fracture (VCF) after spine stereotactic body radiation therapy (SBRT): analysis of predictive factors. *Int J Radat Oncol Biol Phys*. 2012;84:e343–e349.

Chapter 15

Supportive Care in Advanced Renal Cell Carcinoma

Sriram Yennurajalingam

Introduction

In 2014, the expected number of new cases and deaths from renal cell carcinoma (RCC) in the United States will be 63,920 and 13,860, respectively.[1] Improving health-related quality of life (QoL) is an important aspect in the management of RCC because 40%–50% of RCC patients will ultimately develop metastatic disease.[1] Despite advances in treatments such as the use of targeted therapy, many RCC patients suffer from significant physical and psychological symptoms.[2–4] These symptoms impact the QoL of patients and their families. In a recent cross-sectional study of patients with RCC, Harding et al. found that the five most frequent symptoms among patients with localized RCC were irritability (79%), pain (71%), fatigue (71%), worry (71%), and sleep disturbance (64%).[4] Among patients with metastatic disease, the five most frequent symptoms were fatigue (82%), weakness (65%), worry (65%), shortness of breath (53%), and irritability (53%). Various systemic therapies, such as tyrosine kinase inhibitors (TKIs) and antibodies targeting the vascular endothelial growth factor (VEGF) pathway and mammalian target of rapamycin (mTOR) inhibitors, are associated with a higher frequency of symptoms such as pain (eg, stomatitis and hand–foot skin reaction), fatigue, diarrhea, dyspnea, and decreased appetite.[3–7] As a result, all patients with RCC need optimal management of their physical and psychosocial symptoms concurrent with disease-specific treatments throughout the trajectory of their illness. In this chapter, we discuss the assessment and management of the following key symptoms associated with RCC: pain, cancer-related fatigue (CRF), anorexia–cachexia syndrome (ACS), dyspnea, and depression.

Pain

Pain is a complex multidimensional experience in patients with RCC and often has a multifactorial etiology. Pain can arise secondary to direct effects of the tumor at one or multiple metastatic sites or it can be related to cancer treatment. Pain intensity is intrinsically linked to the patient's psychosocial and cultural response to pain, history of addiction, and any underlying cerebral dysfunctions such as delirium.[5] Unrelieved cancer pain impairs mood and interferes with the patient's ability to function and his or her social life.[6]

The management of cancer pain involves routine screening with the use of simple instruments such as the Edmonton symptom assessment scale to evaluate the intensity of pain and its related symptoms such as fatigue, nausea, anxiety, depression, and drowsiness.[5,8] Patients who self-report pain should be investigated for the location, severity, chronicity, and nature (neuropathic, nociceptive, or mixed type) of the pain as well as aggravating and relieving factors.[7] The patient's medication list should include any history of drug abuse and his or her response to previous analgesic treatments. A focused medical history, physical examination, and review of pertinent imaging and laboratory test results should be conducted. Management should then be individualized on the basis of the goals and expectations of the patient and caregivers.

The World Health Organization (WHO) method for providing cancer pain relief, that is, the three-step analgesic ladder approach,[5,9,10] advocates the use of nonopioid analgesics such as acetaminophen and nonsteroidal antiinflammatory drugs (if not contraindicated) for mild pain (first step). If the pain is more severe or not controlled at the first step, escalation to codeine or hydrocodone (second step) or morphine or other strong opioids such as hydromorphone, fentanyl, or oxycodone (third step) should be considered. In addition to stepwise escalation of analgesic strength, the WHO ladder approach includes the principles of "by mouth" (oral administration is preferred over parenteral routes), "by clock" (around-the-clock dosing is used to prevent pain), "for the individual" (treatment plans should be individually tailored), and "attention to detail" (all possible sources of pain and adverse treatment effects should be assessed).

Opioids are the mainstay of cancer pain treatment because a majority of cancer patients have moderate to severe pain. The optimal management of pain using opioids requires periodic reassessment of the pain and its related symptoms in order to determine treatment response and medication side effects. Table 15.1 shows the most commonly prescribed opioids for cancer pain management and their uses, starting dosages, and possible adverse effects.

The most common side effects of opioids are constipation, nausea, and drowsiness. However, opioid-induced neurotoxic side effects such as myoclonus, hallucinations, and delirium are also seen. The side effects are more common in patients with dehydration, infection, renal insufficiency, and liver disease. Therefore, patients with these comorbidities should be closely monitored.

Nonpharmacological approaches such as physical therapy, acupuncture, and counseling or a combined approach can address the multifactorial nature of cancer pain better than the use of analgesics alone. Therefore, for optimal management, a comprehensive assessment and multimodal strategies should always be considered.

Table 15.1 Commonly Prescribed Medications for Management of Cancer-related Symptoms

Drug	Selected Supportive Care Indications	Initial Dose	Adverse Effects
Hydrocodone	Cancer pain	5 mg (in combination with 325 mg with acetaminophen) every hour orally	Nausea, constipation, drowsiness, itching, urinary retention, cognitive impairment, allergic reactions, myoclonus, hallucination, hyperalgesia, allodynia, and liver and renal toxicities due to acetaminophen
Tramadol	Cancer pain	50 mg	Nausea, constipation, drowsiness, itching, urinary retention, cognitive impairment, allergic reactions, myoclonus, hallucination, hyperalgesia, and allodynia
Morphine sulfate	Cancer pain and dyspnea	15 mg every 4 hours (immediate release) orally	
Hydromorphone	Cancer pain and dyspnea	1–2 mg every 4 hours (immediate release) orally	
Oxycodone	Cancer pain and dyspnea	5 mg every 4 hours (immediate release) orally	
Fentanyl	Cancer pain and dyspnea	12 μg/hour transdermally	
Methadone	Cancer pain and dyspnea	2.5–5 mg/day orally	
Dexamethasone	Cancer-related fatigue	Dexamethasone, 8 mg/day for 2 weeks orally	Infection, oral thrush, insomnia, mood swings, myalgia, and elevation of blood glucose

Prolonged use (more than 1 month): gastritis (especially with concurrent use of nonsteroidal antiinflammatory drugs), hiccups, edema, muscle weakness, easy bruising, dizziness, hirsutism, and decreased wound healing |

(Continued)

Table 15.1 (Continued)

Drug	Selected Supportive Care Indications	Initial Dose	Adverse Effects
Methylphenidate	Cancer-related fatigue	5 mg/day orally	Loss of appetite, slurred speech, abnormal behavior, restlessness, Hypertension, tachyarrhythmias, thrombocytopenia, and hallucinations
Modafinil	Cancer-related fatigue	200 mg/day orally	Diarrhea, nausea, dizziness, headache, insomnia, agitation, anxiety, nervousness, and rhinitis. Serious adverse effects include cardiac dysrhythmia, hypertension, and infectious disease
Megestrol acetate	Treatment of cachexia	480–800 mg/day orally	Hypertension, sweating, hot flashes, weight gain, dyspepsia, nausea, vomiting, insomnia, mood swings, and impotence. Serious adverse effects include thrombophlebitis, adrenal insufficiency, and pulmonary embolism
Tricyclic antidepressants • Amitriptyline • Nortryptyline	Depression, neuropathic pain	10–25 mg/day 25 mg/day	Constipation, hypotension, cardiac dysrhythmia, hepatotoxicity, and suicidal thoughts
Selective serotonin reuptake inhibitors • Citalopram • Escitolopram • Fluoxetine • Paroxetine • Sertraline	Depression, panic disorder, and obsessive-compulsive disorder	20 mg/day 10–20 mg/day 20 mg/day 20 mg/day 50 mg/day	Nausea, diarrhea, headache, insomnia, anxiety, anorexia, dizziness, tremor, sweating, and sexual dysfunction

Table 15.1 (Continued)

Drug	Selected Supportive Care Indications	Initial Dose	Adverse Effects
Serotonin–norepinephrine reuptake inhibitors	Depression and neuropathic pain		Nausea, dry mouth, dizziness, excessive sweating, tiredness, difficulty urinating, agitation or anxiety, constipation, insomnia, sexual problems, headache, loss of appetite
• Duloxetine		30 mg/day	
• Venlafaxine		37.5 mg/day	
• Milnacipran		25–50 mg twice a day	
• Mirtazapine		15 mg/day	

Cancer-related Fatigue

CRF is the most common and chronic multidimensional symptom in patients with cancer. The National Comprehensive Cancer Network defines CRF as "a distressing, persistent, subjective sense of physical, emotional, and/or cognitive tiredness or exhaustion related to cancer or cancer treatment that is not proportional to recent activity and that interferes with usual functioning."[11] Various treatments for RCC such as interleukin 2, interferon alpha, and medications that target mTOR, VEGF, or tyrosine kinase receptor result in significantly worse CRF than that associated with the disease itself.[2,7] The exact cause of CRF is not known; however, anemia, electrolyte abnormalities such as hypercalcemia and hyponatremia, infections, endocrine abnormalities such as hypothyroidism and hypogonadism, dysregulation of cytokine production, and hypothalamic–pituitary–adrenergic (HPA) axis dysfunction have been associated with CRF.[11,12]

As in the management of cancer-related pain, screening for CRF using the Edmonton symptom assessment scale should be performed in order to both diagnose and evaluate the intensity, causes, and dimensions of CRF.[12] Investigations should be individualized on the basis of the patient's history and physical examination to confirm the initial diagnosis. Fatigue management should be interdisciplinary and multimodal. Prior studies suggest that physical activity and cognitive behavioral therapy can alleviate CRF.[11] Preliminary studies suggest that among the available pharmacological agents, psychostimulants such as methylphenidate and modafinil may be useful (see Table 15.1). A short course of steroids such as dexamethasone has been suggested for patients with advanced cancer and CRF.[11,12]

Anorexia-Cachexia Syndrome

ACS is a complex syndrome characterized by muscle wasting, loss of body fat, and poor appetite.[12] As with CRF, the exact mechanism of ACS is unknown; however, recent studies point to a proinflammatory state that causes muscle wasting. Abnormalities in neurohormonal function such as elevated cortisol, ghrelin and insulin resistance, low serum testosterone, and sympathetic nervous system activation have been associated with ACS.[13,14] Clinical assessment is by routine screening for patients with a history of involuntary weight loss of >5% of their total body weight within the past 6 months.[13] Factors that contribute to ACS include cancer-related symptoms such as mucositis pain, xerostomia, nausea, dysphagia, depression, and constipation. Other pertinent investigations may include assessing liver function and the levels of serum electrolytes, creatinine, glucose, calcium, testosterone, vitamin B12, vitamin D, thyroid-stimulating hormone, and C-reactive protein. Assessment of metabolism using indirect calorimetry and resting energy expenditure studies helps to detect and treat hypermetabolic states.

Management of ACS includes nutritional counseling, which may include the use of frequent, small, calorie-dense meals. The use of parenteral nutrition is considered only when starvation is a major component, the tumor is slow growing, and the patient is expected to survive at least 6 weeks. Effective management also includes treatment of conditions associated with ACS and pharmacological management using thalidomide, which was useful in preliminary studies, or steroids such as megestrol acetate and dexamethasone (see Table 15.1), which improve appetite but offer no improvement in muscle mass. Preliminary evidence shows additional benefits from melatonin, nonsteroidal antiinflammatory drugs, ghrelin, and ghrelin mimetics. Preliminary evidence also points to the use of exercise (resistance training) for sarcopenia and the benefit of family counseling.[15,16]

Dyspnea

Dyspnea is defined as "a subjective experience of breathing discomfort that consists of qualitatively distinct sensations that vary in intensity. The experience derives from interaction among multiple physiologic, psychological, social, and environmental factors and may induce secondary physiologic and behavioral responses."[17] The frequency of dyspnea varies with the stage of RCC and is seen in approximately 56% of patients with metastatic disease. Dyspnea is debilitating and can significantly impact QoL. Its etiology is multifactorial and usually based on the underlying disease and acuity of onset. The acute causes of dyspnea may include pulmonary embolism, pneumothorax, aspiration, or anxiety. Subacute causes are pneumonia, pleural effusion, pericardial effusion, superior vena cava obstruction, anemia, and radiation-induced pneumonitis. Chronic causes include radiation-induced fibrosis, chemotherapy-induced pulmonary fibrosis, renal failure, and cardiomyopathy.

The assessment of dyspnea should routinely include screening for severity using a visual analogue scale or numerical rating scale such as the Edmonton symptom assessment scale. Further assessment in patients with moderate to severe dyspnea may include investigations of onset, duration, pattern (incidental or continuous), and associated symptoms such as anxiety, depression, cough, chest pain, wheezing, chest tightness, hemoptysis, and weight loss/gain. Physical examinations (such as those measuring heart rate, respiratory rate, oxygen saturation at rest and after a 6-minute walk, jugular venous pressure, and breath sounds) and laboratory tests (including complete blood count, chest x-ray, pulmonary function tests, and echocardiography) should be guided by the patient's history.[18]

Various medications benefit patients with significant dyspnea. Opioids are commonly used in the management of dyspnea (see Table 15.1), and several studies suggest improvement of dyspnea with opioids (oral or systemic routes). Other medications in appropriate settings may include bronchodilators, corticosteroids, diuretics, antibiotics, and anticoagulants.

Nonpharmacological measures such as oxygen therapy in patients with hypoxemia and noninvasive ventilation should be considered in select situations. In advanced cancer patients, if short trials of these measures do not improve dyspnea, they should be discontinued. Other helpful nonpharmacological measures include the use of a hand fan with cool air blowing onto the face, chest wall percussive vibration, mechanical devices, and pulmonary rehabilitation. In all patients, relaxation techniques, psychosocial support, and activity modification can be beneficial.

Surgical interventions for dyspnea may include thoracentesis (for pleural effusion) or the placement of a chest tube (for pneumothorax) or metallic stents (for airway obstruction).

Depression

Depression is defined as a persistent low mood, or anhedonia, that lasts for 2 weeks or longer and is accompanied by at least four of the following symptoms: sleep disruption, changes in weight or appetite, psychomotor retardation or agitation, fatigue or loss of energy, feelings of worthlessness or excessive guilt, diminished ability to think or concentrate, and recurrent thoughts of death or suicidal ideation. Depression may contribute to progression of RCC via multifactorial mechanisms. Recent evidence points to the central role of dysregulation of proinflammatory cytokines and the HPA axis.[19] In patients with RCC, depression may be a result of the disease and/or a treatment-related side effect (eg, in the case of interferon therapy). Depression is diagnosed using a single-item evaluation such as, "Are you depressed most of the time?" or using other reliable tools such as the Centers for Epidemiologic Studies-Depression or hospital anxiety depression scale. The fifth edition of the *Diagnostic and Statistical Manual of Mental Disorders* further subclassifies patients with severe forms of depression as having major depressive or bipolar disorders. Patients with advanced cancer usually have milder forms of depression such as adjustment disorder with depressed mood, dysthymia, and recurrent brief depression.

Depressed mood occurs frequently in patients with cancer, and periods of sadness are expected when dealing with cancer and treatment. However, if the depressed mood persists and causes pervasive interference with daily function or accompanies other symptoms of major depression, treatment should be considered. Management should include psychotherapy and antidepressant medication (see Table 15.1). Pharmacological management is determined by the patient's prognosis, drug interactions, and medication side effects. Selective serotonin reuptake inhibitors, serotonin–norepinephrine reuptake inhibitors, and psychostimulants are used most frequently because of their tolerable side-effect profiles. The combination of antidepressants with psychotherapy has been found to be more effective than either treatment alone. Supportive psychotherapy that allows patients to express worries, fears, and concerns as well as validation of and support for the patient can also be helpful. Other types of recommended psychotherapy include cognitive behavioral, family, interpersonal, and mindfulness-based therapies.[20,21]

Summary

Patients with RCC suffer from various physical and psychological symptoms including pain, fatigue, ACS, dyspnea, and depression due to the disease and its treatments. These adversely affect a patient's QoL. An interdisciplinary approach that includes various supportive care strategies should be used concurrently with cancer-specific therapy to provide quality cancer care.

References

1. American Cancer Society: Cancer Facts and Figures 2014. Atlanta, Ga: American Cancer Society, 2014. http://www.cancer.org/acs/groups/content/@research/documents/webcontent/acspc-042151.pdf Last accessed, May 12, 2014.2.

2. Turner JS, Cheung EM, George J, Quinn DI. Pain management, supportive and palliative care in patients with renal cell carcinoma. *BJU Intl.* 2007;99(5b):1305–1312.

3. Lambea J, Hinojo C, Lainez N, Lázaro M, León L, Rodríguez A, et al. Quality of life and supportive care for patients with metastatic renal cell carcinoma. *Cancer Metastasis Rev.* 2012;31(1):33–39.

4. Harding G, et al. Symptom burden among patients with renal cell carcinoma (RCC): content for a symptom index. *Health Qual Life Outcomes.* 2007;5(1):34.

5. Hui D, Bruera E: A Personalized Approach to Assessing and Managing Pain in Patients With Cancer. Journal of Clinical Oncology, 2014

6. Cella D. Beyond traditional outcomes: improving quality of life in patients with renal cell carcinoma. *Oncologist.* 2011;16 (suppl 2):23–31.

7. Méndez-Vidal MJ, Martínez Ortega E, Montesa Pino A, Pérez Valderrama B, Viciana R. Management of adverse events of targeted therapies in normal and special patients with metastatic renal cell carcinoma. *Cancer Metastasis Rev.* 2012;31(1):19–27.

8. Bruera E, Kuehn N, Miller MJ, Selmser P, Macmillan K. The Edmonton Symptom Assessment System (ESAS): a simple method for the assessment of palliative care patients. *J Palliat Care.* 1991;7 (2):6.

9. Bruera E, Kim HN. Cancer pain. *JAMA.* 2003;290:2476–2479.

10. WHO. *Cancer Pain Relief and Palliative Care: Report of a WHO Expert Committee* Geneva, Switzerland: World Health Organization; 1990.

11. Berger AM, Abernethy AP, Atkinson A, Barsevick AM, Breitbart WS, Cella D, et al. Cancer-related fatigue. *J Natl Compr Canc Netw.* 2010;8(8):904–931.

12. Yennurajalingam S, Bruera E. Palliative management of fatigue at the close of life. *JAMA.* 2007;297(3):295–304.

13. Fearon K, Strasser F, Anker SD, Bosaeus I, Bruera E, Fainsinger RL, et al. Definition and classification of cancer cachexia: an international consensus. *Lancet Oncol.,* 2011;12(5):489–495.

14. Tisdale MJ. Molecular pathways leading to cancer cachexia. *Physiology.* 2005;20(5):340–348.

15. Blum D, Omlin A, Baracos VE, Solheim TS, Tan BH, Stone P, et al. Cancer cachexia: A systematic literature review of items and domains associated with involuntary weight loss in cancer. *Crit Rev Oncol Hematol.* 2011;80(1):114–144.

16. Yavuzsen T, Davis MP, Walsh D, LeGrand S, Lagman R, et al. Systematic review of the treatment of cancer-associated anorexia and weight loss. *J Clin Oncol.* 2005;23(33):8500–8511.

17. American Thoracic Society. Dyspnea: mechanisms, assessment, and management: a consensus statement. *Am J Respir Crit Care Med.* 2001;163:951–957.

18. Viola R, Kiteley C, Lloyd NS, Mackay JA, Wilson J, Wong RKS. The management of dyspnea in cancer patients: a systematic review. *Support Care Cancer.* 2008;16:329–337.

19. Miller AH, Ancoli-Israel S, Bower JE, Capuron L, Irwin MR., et al. Neuroendocrine-immune mechanisms of behavioral comorbidities in patients with cancer. J Clin Oncol. 2008;26(6):971–982.

20. Wilson KG, Chochinov HM, Skirko MG, Allard P, Chary S, Gagnon PR, Macmillan K, et al. Depression and anxiety disorders in palliative cancer care. *J Pain Symptom Manage.* 2007;33(2):118–129.

21. Cipriani A, Furukawa TA, Salanti G, Geddes JR, Higgins JP, Churchill R, et al. Comparative efficacy and acceptability of 12 new-generation antidepressants: A multiple-treatments meta-analysis. *Lancet.* 2009;373:746–758.

Chapter 16

Integrative Medicine in the Management of Renal Cell Carcinoma

Alejandro Chaoul, Gabriel Lopez, Richard Lee, M. Kay Garcia, and Lorenzo Cohen

Introduction

Complementary and alternative medicine (CAM) approaches of care have gained increasing acceptance among those practicing conventional Western medicine. With an increasing number of CAM offerings, patients are in need of guidance as to how to navigate the available information in order to make informed decisions about their use. Developing an integrative care plan requires a thoughtful, evidence-based, and safe approach to including nonconventional CAM therapies with conventional disease-directed therapeutics. An integrative approach provides patients, from diagnosis through survivorship, with a comprehensive system of care to help meet their needs. The majority of cancer patients are either using complementary medicines or want to know more about them, so it is incumbent on those within the conventional medical system to provide appropriate education and evidenced-based clinical services. The clinical model for integrative care requires a patient-centered approach with attention to patient concerns and enhanced communication skills. In addition, it is essential that conventional and nonconventional practitioners work together to develop a comprehensive, integrative care plan that will deliver the best medical care by using all appropriate treatment modalities in a safe manner to achieve optimal clinical outcomes.

Definitions: Alternative, Complementary, Integrative

The US National Center for Complementary and Alternative Medicine (NCCAM) defines CAM as "a group of diverse medical and healthcare systems, practices, and products that are not normally considered to be part of conventional medicine."[1] NCCAM recently reclassified CAM therapies into three broad categories: natural products, mind and body medicine, and other complementary medicine practices that are approaches that do not fit neatly into either of the other two categories (Table 16.1).

It is important to recognize the distinction between alternative, complementary, and integrative medicine.[2] Alternative medicine is the use of a nonconventional modality for which there is no scientific evidence of efficacy in place of conventional medicine. Complementary medicine is an approach that combines conventional treatment with CAM or nonconventional

Table 16.1 Complementary Health Approaches

Complementary and Alternative Medicine Subcategories	Examples
Natural products	Dietary supplements • Herbal medicines (botanicals) • Vitamins • Minerals • Probiotics
Mind and body practices, includes the former categories of manipulative and body-based practices and energy therapies	Meditation Yoga Qi gong Tai chi Relaxation techniques • Breathing exercises • Guided imagery • Progressive muscle relaxation Hypnotherapy Energy therapies • Healing touch • Reiki • Magnet therapy Acupuncture Massage therapy Spinal manipulation • Chiropractic • Osteopathic • Physical therapy Movement therapies • Feldenkrais • Pilates • Alexander technique
Other complementary health approaches	Whole medical systems • Traditional healers • Ayurvedic medicine • Traditional Chinese medicine • Homeopathy • Naturopathy

http://nccam.nih.gov/health/whatiscam. Accessed May 11, 2014.

therapies for which there may or may not exist scientific evidence of safety and effectiveness. Integrative medicine seeks to merge conventional medicine and complementary therapies in a manner that is comprehensive, personalized, evidence based, and safe in order to achieve optimal health and healing.

Complementary and Alternative Medicine and Symptom Management

Routine assessment for interest in and prior use of CAM is critical to the ongoing care of patients and for ensuring the highest quality of care.[3] A collaborative approach that involves the patient's oncology team and colleagues in integrative medicine, palliative care, pain management, psychiatry, and rehabilitation can more effectively meet patient needs. For those seeking integrative medicine approaches for the management of their symptoms, this assessment is critical. CAM approaches can be incorporated into the healthcare plan from diagnosis, through active treatment, survivorship, and end-of-life care. A personalized symptom management strategy that uses an evidence-based application of conventional and nonconventional therapies can help to improve quality of life (QoL) and optimize treatment outcomes.

Communicating about Complementary and Alternative Medicine

Research indicates that neither adult nor pediatric cancer patients receive sufficient information or discuss CAM therapies with physicians, pharmacists, nurses, or CAM practitioners.[4] Using a receptive, nonjudgmental approach when asking patients about CAM use is an important first step to developing an integrative care plan. Most patients do not bring up the topic of CAM because no one asks; thus, patients may believe it is unimportant. It is estimated that 38%–60% of patients with cancer used complementary approaches without informing their healthcare team.[5] This lack of discussion is of concern because biologically based therapies (such as herbs) may interact with cancer treatments. Patients are commonly unaware of differences between the US Food and Drug Administration (FDA) approval process for medications and the limited extent of regulation for dietary supplements under the Dietary Supplement Health and Education Act of 1994.[6] Supplements under this legislation are exempt from the same scrutiny the FDA imposes on medications; these supplements are not intended to treat, prevent, or cure diseases and should be labeled with this statement.

The common belief by patients that "natural" means safe needs to be addressed with education. Some herbs and supplements have been associated with drug interactions,[7] increased cancer risk,[8] and organ toxicity.[9] Existing research suggests that the majority of cancer patients desire communication with their doctors about CAM.[10] If the issue of CAM arises, clinicians need to develop an empathic communication strategy.[11] The strategy needs to balance clinical objectivity and creation of a therapeutic

Table 16.2 Recommended Web Sites for Evidence-based Resources

Organization/Web Site	Address/URL
American Cancer Society	www.cancer.org/treatment/ treatmentsandsideeffects/ complementaryandalternativemedicine/ index
Cochrane Review Organization	www.cochrane.org
Memorial Sloan-Kettering Cancer Center Integrative Medicine Service	www.mskcc.org/aboutherbs
National Center for Complementary and Alternative Medicine	nccam.nih.gov
Natural Medicines Comprehensive Database	www.naturaldatabase.com
Natural Standard	www.naturalstandard.com
National Cancer Institute Office of Cancer Complementary and Alternative Medicine	www.cancer.gov/cam
University of Texas M. D. Anderson Cancer Center Integrative Medicine Program	mdanderson.org/Integrativemed

alliance. Patients need reliable information on CAM from reliable resources, with adequate time to discuss this information with their oncologists (Table 16.2).

Complementary and Alternative Medicine Modalities

Natural products; mind and body approaches including meditation, yoga, massage, acupuncture; and music therapy are nonconventional therapies that are commonly used in a variety of healthcare settings. See Table 16.2.

Natural Products

Natural products include a variety of substances such as herbs, vitamins, minerals, probiotics, and extracts. Biologically based CAM therapies such as natural products have the potential to cause harm. There is also great interest in investigating how these substances can be used safely along with conventional treatments to improve outcomes. Issues to consider when discussing natural products include quality control, metabolic interactions, treatment interactions, organ toxicity, and cancer growth.[12,13]

Mind and Body Therapies

There are a number of reasons why it is important for cancer patients to manage stress, not the least of which is to help improve QoL. In addition, there is emerging research that shows that depression, independent of disease severity, is associated with increased mortality.[14] A recent study of patients with stage IV renal cell carcinoma (RCC) found that depressive symptoms were associated with decreased survival and this was partially mediated through inflammatory signaling.[15]

There are a number of ways to help address stress in cancer patients. Mind and body therapies include practices such as relaxation, yoga, meditation, tai chi, qi gong, hypnosis, imagery, biofeedback, cognitive-behavioral therapies, group support, and spirituality. Other mind–body approaches include expressive arts therapies (eg, art, music, or dance), body manipulation practices (eg, massage and acupuncture), and energy medicine (eg, Reiki and healing touch therapies).

Ernst et al. examined changes in the state of the evidence for mind–body therapies for various medical conditions between 2000 and 2005. They found that over that period, maximal evidence had appeared for the use of relaxation techniques for anxiety, hypertension, insomnia, and nausea due to chemotherapy.[16]

Research examining yoga, tai chi, and meditation incorporated into cancer care suggests that these practices help improve QoL through improved mood, sleep quality, physical functioning, and overall well-being.[17] Mind–body practitioners who are experienced working with cancer patients can provide guidance to help patients engage safely in practices such as meditation, yoga, and tai chi. Mind–body approaches can be incorporated successfully with more conventional therapies such as psychotherapy, cognitive behavioral therapy, and psychotropic medications.

Music Therapy

Music therapy is a mind–body practice that uses music (music making, songwriting, singing, listening) in a prescriptive manner for nonmusical goals including improving QoL.[18] Trained music therapists choose a music approach most appropriate to help patients achieve a desired result. Evidence suggests music therapy can help with management of mood disturbances, including anxiety.[19] An integrative medicine practitioner can help identify those patients most likely to benefit from consultation with a music therapist.

Massage

As a manipulative touch-based therapy, massage can benefit cancer patients when it is performed by individuals who have an awareness of their special needs.[20] A massage therapist with special training in oncology massage is the best equipped to safely deliver the massage. Risk of bruising, bleeding, or injury can be minimized by careful application of pressure, avoiding massage into the deep tissue or bone in selected patients. Areas that have recently had surgery or radiation should be avoided.

Research to date suggests that massage is helpful at relieving pain, anxiety, fatigue, and distress and at increasing relaxation.[21] Benefit on mood and pain relief is limited to the more immediate effect of massage, with no current studies demonstrating long-term relief.[22] Massage provided by caregivers may offer a unique opportunity for interaction between patient and caregiver that can help enhance well-being of both.[23]

Acupuncture

Many cancer patients use acupuncture to help with symptom management. In 1997, the National Institutes of Health published a consensus statement supporting its use for postoperative and chemotherapy-related nausea/vomiting and some types of pain.[24] Studies have since supported this decision, although scientifically rigorous research is still greatly needed to confirm benefits, especially when used to help with other symptoms such as dry mouth, hot flashes, and fatigue.[25,26] The underlying biological mechanisms of acupuncture are not well understood but are believed to include enhanced conduction of bioelectromagnetic signals, activation of opioid systems, and activation of the autonomic and central nervous systems, which results in the release of various neurotransmitters and neurohormones.[27] Based on the theory of traditional Chinese medicine, acupuncture is said to help to regulate the flow of *qi* (vital energy).[27]

The most common form of acupuncture involves the insertion of small needles into the skin at specific points on the body. For some patients, acupressure may be used, which involves applying heat or pressure to acupoints instead of puncturing the skin. When performed correctly, acupuncture is a safe, minimally invasive procedure with few side effects.[28,29]

Nutrition and Exercise

Growing evidence supports the important role of nutrition and physical activity in the health of cancer patients. These factors have been correlated with improved clinical outcomes. [30,31] An integrative care plan is not complete without a personalized discussion regarding a patient's individual dietary needs and physical activity goals.

Diet and Nutrition

Addressing a patient's individual dietary needs is crucial, especially with the prevalence of obesity. The American Cancer Society's (ACS) Prevention Study "showed significant increases in cancer occurrence in people who are the most overweight" and in certain cancers, including kidney cancer, the link is stronger.[32] Obesity has been cited as one of the top risk factors for RCC, and as the authors of this study mentioned, "identifying risk factors offers an opportunity for targeted education and intervention."[33] Patients are flooded with a number of dietary approaches to follow and need guidance. Some of these choices may be harmful during active treatment, leading to poor outcomes. ACS diet guidelines suggest at least five servings of vegetables and fruit per day. A large US cohort study found that eating a diet rich in fiber was associated with a significantly lower risk of RCC.[34] Diets labeled as "anti-cancer" that are composed strictly of raw foods, juiced fruits and vegetables, animal protein sources, or alkaline foods have no evidence to support their use and may be harmful during active treatment, lacking the nutrients necessary for healing and recovery. Referral to a dietician can help patients and survivors identify how to best meet their nutritional needs. As a general approach, a diet rich in fruits, vegetables, whole grains, and lean meats with an avoidance of processed foods can be part of a healthy lifestyle.

Exercise

Exercise can be important to patients receiving active treatment as well as survivors, helping to improve physical function and QoL.[35] Regular exercise during cancer therapies such as chemotherapy or radiation has the potential

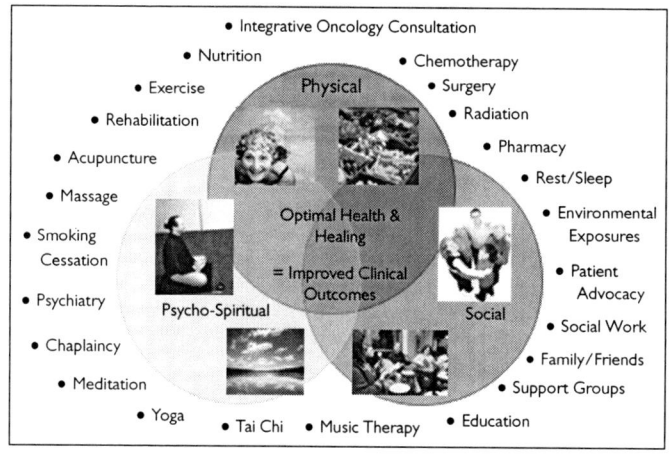

Figure 16.1 Our Integrative Medicine Model based on George Engel's BioPsychoSocial model.[38] George L. Engel, The Need for a New Medical Model: A Challenge for Biomedicine, Science, New Series, Vol. 196, No. 4286 (Apr. 8, 1977), pp. 129–136

to decrease treatment-related fatigue.[36] ACS guidelines for cancer prevention recommend avoidance of sedentary behavior, encouraging 150 minutes of moderate physical activity spread throughout the week.[30] Trinh and colleagues looked specifically at exercise in kidney cancer survivors and found that more than half of kidney cancer survivors are completely inactive and only a quarter are meeting physical activity guidelines.[37] Specialists in cancer rehabilitation can help develop an individualized, safe, and structured program of exercise for patients and survivors.

Summary

Integrative oncology is an expanding discipline that holds tremendous promise for additional treatment and symptom control options. An integrative approach provides patients, from diagnosis through survivorship, with a comprehensive system of care to help meet their needs. An integrative, interdisciplinary approach that advocates open communication between conventional and nonconventional healthcare providers can help patients better meet their goals in a safe manner (Figure 16.1).

References

1. National Center for Complementary/Alternative Medicine (NCCAM) of the National Institutes of Health. Are You Considering Complementary Medicine? December 2006; last updated March 2013. NCCAM Pub. No. D339. Available from http://nccam.nih.gov/health/decisions/consideringcam.htm. Accessed May 11, 2014.

2. Deng G, Cassileth B. Complementary or alternative medicine in cancer care-myths and realities. *Nat Rev Clin Oncol.* 2013; Nov;10(11):656–664. doi: 10.1038/nrclinonc.2013.125. Epub 2013 July 30.

3. Frenkel M, Cohen, L. Peterson, N., Palmer, L. Swint, K., Bruera, E. Integrative medicine consultation service in a comprehensive cancer center: findings and outcomes. *Integr Cancer Ther.* 2010;9(3):276–283.

4. Oneschuk D, et al. The use of complementary medications by cancer patients attending an outpatient pain and symptom clinic. *J Palliat Care.* 1998;14(4):21–26.

5. Navo MA, et al., An assessment of the utilization of complementary and alternative medication in women with gynecologic or breast malignancies. *J Clin Oncol.* 2004;22(4):671–677.

6. 103rd Congress. Dietary Supplement Health and Education Act of 1994 (DSHEA). *Public Law.* 103–417. 10-25-1994.

7. Ulbricht C, Chao W, Costa D, et al. Clinical evidence of herb-drug interactions: a systematic review by the natural standard research collaboration. *Curr Drug Metab.* 2008;9(10):1063–1120.

8. Klein EA, et al. Vitamin E and the risk of prostate cancer: the Selenium and Vitamin E Cancer Prevention Trial (SELECT). *JAMA.* 2011;306(14):1549–1556.

9. Mazzanti G, et al. Hepatotoxicity from green tea: a review of the literature and two unpublished cases. *Eur J Clin Pharmacol.* 2009;65:331–341.

10. Verhoef MJ, White MA, Doll R. Cancer patients' expectations of the role of family physicians in communication about complementary therapies. *Cancer Prev Control.* 1999;3(3):181–187.

11. Berk LB. Primer on integrative oncology. *Hematol Oncol Clin North Am.* 2006;20(1):213–231.

12. OCCAM. Talking About Complementary and Alternative Medicine With Your Health Care Provider: A Workbook and Tips. http://cam.cancer.gov/talking_about_cam.html. Accessed May 11, 2014.

13. Grabowsky JA. Drug interactions and the pharmacist: focus on everolimus. *Ann Pharmacother.* 2013;47(7–8):1055–1063.

14. Satin JR, Linden W, Phillips MJ. Depression as a predictor of disease progression and mortality in cancer patients: a meta-analysis. *Cancer.* 2009;115:5349–5361.

15. Cohen L, Cole SW, Sood AK, et al. Depressive symptoms and cortisol rhythmicity predict survival in patients with renal cell carcinoma: role of inflammatory signaling. *PLoS One.* 2012;7(8):e42324.

16. Ernst E, Pittler MH, Wider B, et al. Mind-body therapies: are the trial data getting stronger? *Altern Ther Health Med.* 2007;13(5):62–64.

17. Mustian KM, Sprod LK, Janelsins M, et al. Multicenter, randomized controlled trial of yoga for sleep quality among cancer survivors. *J Clin Oncol.* 2013 Sep 10;31(26):3233–3241. doi: 10.1200/JCO.2012.43.7707. Epub 2013 Aug 12.

18. Hilliard, Russell E. The effects of music therapy on the quality and length of life of people diagnosed with terminal cancer. *J Music Ther.* 2003;XL2:113–137.

19. Richardson M, Babiak-Vazquez AE, Frenkel MA. Music therapy in a comprehensive cancer center. *J Soc Integr Oncol.* 2008;6(2):76–81.

20. Collinge W, MacDonald G, Walton T. Massage in supportive cancer care. *Semin Oncol Nurs.* 2012;28(1):45–54.

21. Russell NC, et al., Role of massage therapy in cancer care. *J Altern Complement Med.* 2008;14(2):209–214.

22. Kutner JS, et al. Massage therapy versus simple touch to impove pain and mood in patient with advanced cancer: a randomized trial. *Ann Intern Med.* 2008;149(6):369–379.

23. Collinge W, Kahn J, Walton T, et al. Touch, caring, and cancer: randomized controlled trial of a multimedia caregiver education program. *Support Care Cancer.* 2013;21(5):1405–1414.

24. National Institutes of Health Consensus Panel. *Acupuncture: NIH Consensus Development Conference Statement,* Nov. 3–5, 1997;15(5):1–34.

25. Garcia MK, McQuade J, Haddad R, et al. Systematic review of acupuncture in cancer care: a synthesis of the evidence. *J Clin Oncol.* 2013;31(7):952–960.

26. Acupuncture PDQ. National Cancer Institute. http://www.cancer.gov/can certopics/pdq/cam/acupuncture/patient/page2. Last modified June 18, 2013.

27. Helms JM. *Acupuncture Energetics: A Clinical Approach for Physicians. Berkeley.* Berkeley: Medical Acupuncture Publishers; 1997; 20–42.

28. Ernst E, White AR. Prospective studies of the safety of acupuncture: a systematic review. *Am J Med.* 2001;110(6):481–485.

29. Filshie J. Safety aspects of acupuncture in palliative care. *Acupunct Med.* 2001;19(2):117–122.

30. Kushi CL, et al. American Cancer Society Guidelines on Nutrition and Physical Activity for Cancer Prevention: Reducing the Risk of Cancer With Healthy Food Choices and Physical Activity. *CA Cancer J Clin.* 2012;62:30–67.

31. Rock CL, et al. Nutrition and physical activity guidelines for cancer survivors. *CA Cancer J Clin.* 2012;62:242–274.

32. American Cancer Society. The obesity-cancer connection, and what we can know about it. February 28, 2013 http://www.cancer.org/cancer/news/expert-voices/post/2013/02/28/the-obesity-cancer-connection-and-what-we-can-do-about-it.aspx

33. Macleod LC, Hotaling JM, Wright JL, et al. Risk factors for renal cell carcinoma in the VITAL Study. *J Urol.* 2013 Nov;190(5):1657–1661. doi: 10.1016/j.juro.2013.04.130. Epub 2013 May 9..

34. Daniel CR, Park Y, Chow WH, Graubard BI, Hollenbeck AR, Sinha R. Intake of fiber and fiber-rich plant foods is associated with a lower risk of renal cell carcinoma in a large US cohort. *Am J Clin Nutr.* 2013;97(5):1036–1043.

35. Mishra SI, Scherer RW, Snyder C, Geigle PM, Berlanstein DR, Topaloglu O. Exercise interventions on health-related quality of life for people with cancer during active treatment (review). *Cochrane Database Sys Rev.* 2012, issue 8.

36. Cramp F, Byron-Daniel J. Exercise for the management of cancer-related fatigue in adults. *Cochrane Database Syst Rev.* 2012;Nov 14;11: CD006145.

37. Trinh L, Plotnikoff RC, Rhodes RE, North S, Courneya KS. Correlates of physical activity in a population-based sample of kidney cancer survivors: An application of the theory of planned behavior. *Intl J Behav Nutr Phys Act.* 2012; 9(96). doi:10.1186/1479-5868-9-96

38. George L. Engel, The Need for a New Medical Model: A Challenge for Biomedicine, *Science,* New Series, Vol. 196, No. 4286 (Apr. 8, 1977), 129–136.

Chapter 17

Emerging Therapies and Future Directions in Renal Cell Carcinoma

George K. Philips and Michael B. Atkins

Introduction

Given the limitations of current therapies either used alone or in combination, new treatment approaches with an improved therapeutic index are needed for patients with advanced renal cell carcinoma (RCC). Such strategies will need to be based on a deeper understanding of the mechanisms that underlie vascular endothelial growth factor (VEGF) and mammalian target of rapamycin (mTOR) pathway inhibitor and immunotherapy refractoriness or acquired resistance and the development of novel agents that target these and other pathways. Several of the more promising approaches are described below and summarized in Table 17.1.

Inhibitors of Acquired Resistance to Vascular Endothelial Growth Factor Receptor Tyrosine Kinase Inhibitors

Current research suggests that acquired resistance to VEGF receptor (VEGFR) tyrosine kinase inhibitors (TKIs) is frequently mediated through the activation of alternative signaling pathways that restore tumor perfusion (referred to as "angiogenic escape"). Factors that have been shown to contribute to the angiogenic escape associated with VEGFR TKI resistance include upregulation of the expression of angiopoeitins, activin-like kinase-1 (ALK-1) receptor, sphingosine kinase, cMet, interleukin 8 (IL-8), and loss of P53 function. Inhibitors of several of these pathways have been explored preclinically, and some have entered clinical investigation in patients with advanced RCC. Principal results of these experiments and early clinical trials are described in this section.

Angiopoietins

The angiopoietins, Ang-1 and Ang-2, specific ligands for the endothelial-specific tyrosine kinase receptors Tie-1 and Tie-2, are thought to play a key role in

Table 17.1 Selected Novel Targets and Investigational Agents for Treating Renal Cell Carcinoma

Novel Targets	Target Class	Agent	Agent Type	Reference
Angiopoietin/Tie-2 axis(angiogenesis)	Angiopoietins	AMG-386 (trebaninib)	Anti-angiopoietin peptibody	4, 5
ALK-1 (angiogenesis)	Transforming growth factor receptor family	Dalantercept	Soluble fusion protein of ALK-1 and human immunoglobulin-G1 Fc, ligand trap for BMP9 and 10	clinicaltrials.gov NCT00996957 NCT01642082
Sphingosine-1-phosphate (angiogenesis)	Sphingolipid, signaling molecule	Sonepcizumab (LT1009)	Humanized sphingomab antibody	19 clinicaltrials.gov NCT01762033
Human double minute 2 (p53 modulation and angiogenesis regulation)	E3 ubiquitin ligase	JNJ-26854165, RO5045337, MK-8242	Small-molecule mdm2 inhibitors	clinicaltrials.gov NCT00555933 NCT00623870
c-MET (tumorigenesis, angiogenesis, bone metabolism)	Receptor tyrosine kinase (proto-oncogene)	Cabozantinib (XL184), onartuzumab (MetMAb), ARQ 197, foretinib	Small-molecule dual kinase inhibitor of MET and vascular endothelial growth factor receptor2, monovalent antibody	11, 12
IL-8(angiogenesis)	Chemokine of CXC family	Preclinical	IL-8 antibody	24
Hypoxia-inducible factor-2 alpha (tumorigenesis, angiogenesis)	Basic helix–loop–helix family of transcription factors	None	None	28
mTORC1/2 and PI3K(angiogenesis, acquired resistance to TORC1 inhibitors)	PI3K-related kinase protein family	BEZ235, BKM120, GDC-0980	Dual mTORC1/2 and/or PI3K small-molecule inhibitors	34, 35 www.clinicaltrials.gov NCT01283048 NCT01442090

Polybromo 1 and *BAP1* (tumor suppressor genes)	Chromatin remodeling complexes regulation transcription; *BAP1* codes for a nuclear deubiquitinase	None	None	
Neurofibromin 2 (Merlin) and Hippo pathway (tumor suppressor genes)	Growth regulatory signaling pathways (pro-proliferative, anti-apoptotic)	None	None	41
PD1 / PD-L1 pathwayCTLA-4	Immune checkpoints	Nivolumab, MPDL3280A	Antibodies to PD1 or PD-L1	

ALK-1, activin-like kinase-1; *BAP1*, BRCA1-associated protein-1; IL-8, interlukin-8; mTORC, mTOR complex; PI3K, phosphatidyl inositol 3 kinase; CTLA-4, Cytotoxic T-Lymphocyte Antigen 4.

blood vessel maturation and integrity. Ang-1 and Ang-2 are highly expressed by the endothelial cells of many tumors and co-promote neoplastic angiogenesis along with VEGF. The Ang/Tie-2 pathway is involved in both basal angiogenesis in response to hypoxia in RCC and in vascular stability in the setting of VEGF blockade.[1,2] In mouse tumors and human tumor xenografts, a bispecific Ang-2–VEGF-A monoclonal antibody led to potent inhibition of tumor-selective angiogenesis, an enhanced vessel maturation phenotype, and inhibition of hematogeneous metastases.[3]

AMG-386 (trebaninib) is an anti-angiopoietin peptibody (peptide-Fc fusion protein) that can disrupt the angiopoietin/Tie-2 axis. Since VEGF and Ang-2 cooperate to promote angiogenesis, the simultaneous use of trebaninib with anti-VEGF agents has the potential to intensify anti-angiogenic pressure in RCC. Clinical results of combination VEGFR TKI and trebaninib therapy have been mixed. A randomized phase 2 trial of sorafenib plus either trebaninib at 10 or 3mg/kg weekly or placebo in patients with advanced RCC showed a higher objective response rate (ORR;38% and 37% versus 25%) in the trebaninib-containing arms; however, there was no significant impact on median progression-free survival (PFS).[4] Further, patients receiving sorafenib + placebo who crossed over to sorafenib + open-label trebaninib at 10 mg/kg weekly had an ORR of 3%, indicating that the addition of trebaninib could not overcome the acquired resistance to sorafenib. However, in a phase 2 study of sunitinib plus sequential cohorts of trebaninib at 10 mg/kg or 15 mg/kg, the PFS was 13.9 months in the low-dose cohort and more than16 months in the high-dose cohort.[5] The overall response rates were 58% and 59%, respectively, suggesting enhanced antitumor activity for the combination. Additionally, this apparent beneficial effect was achieved without significant additional toxicity, as virtually all side effects were attributable to sunitinib. The explanation for the potential improvement in median PFS for trebaninib when combined with sunitinib relative to sorafenib is not clear.

c-MET and Hepatocyte Growth Factor—Cabozantinib

Activation of c-MET in RCC has been linked to *VHL* loss as well as hypoxia.[6,7] Higher expression of c-MET in RCC tumor specimens has been associated with higher tumor grade and clinical stage and was also found to be an independent predictor of poor overall survival.[8] In human tumor xenograft models, c-MET expression was found to be significantly higher in endothelial cells than in tumor cells and appeared to induce the development of resistance to VEGF-targeted therapy through maintenance of an alternate angiogenic pathway.[9] Hepatocyte growth factor (HGF), the ligand for c-MET, is expressed in higher concentrations in VEGF pathway inhibitor-resistant tumors, supporting a role for the c-MET/HGF pathway in the acquired resistance to anti-angiogenic therapy. Furthermore, a combination of sunitinib and a selective c-Met inhibitor exhibited synergistic inhibition of RCC tumor growth in resistant tumors.[9]

Cabozantinib (XL184) is a small-molecule kinase inhibitor that targets both MET and VEGFR2 as well as a number of other potentially relevant receptor tyrosine kinases, including RET, KIT, AXL, and FLT3. In a human tumor xenograft model, cabozantinib disrupted tumor vasculature, increased tumor hypoxia 13-fold, promoted tumor and endothelial cell death, and inhibited tumor growth in a dose-dependent manner.[10] Cabozantinib has activity in a wide variety of human tumors and is approved for the treatment of medullary thyroid cancer.

In 25 previously treated patients (the majority had VEGF-targeted therapy and 50% had three or more prior therapies) with metastatic RCC given cabozantinib up to 140 mg daily, 7 (28%) had an objective response and 13 (52%) had stable disease;[11] the median PFS was 14.7 months. Three of four patients with bone metastases had a response and two had effective palliation of bone pain. These encouraging preliminary data have led to initiation of randomized trials of cabozantinib in the first-line setting (phase 2 versus sunitinib; NCT01835158) and after resistance to a VEGFR TKI (phase 3 versus everolimus; NCT01865747). A variety of other c-MET small-molecule receptor tyrosine kinase inhibitors and antibodies to HGF or c-MET are also undergoing clinical investigation.[12] These agents are now likely to be explored both as single agents and in combination with VEGF-targeted therapy in patients with advanced RCC. A special role for c-MET inhibitors in papillary RCC may also emerge because of the critical role of activating c-MET mutations in that disease.

Activin-like Kinase-1: Dalantercept

The transforming growth factor-beta (TGF-β) receptor family members ALK-1 and endoglin (ENG) and their ligands, bone morphogenetic protein (BMP) 9 and 10, appear to play roles in vascular formation that are distinct from VEGF. Patients with genetic alterations in ALK-1 or ENG develop hereditary hemorrhagic telangiectasia. The role of ALK-1 in angiogenesis is complex and context dependent. However, emerging data suggest that while VEGF is critical for early endothelial proliferation and sprouting, ALK-1 has a major role in the development of mature, functional vascular beds.

ALK-1 inhibitors under development include ACE-041 (dalantercept) and PF-03446962. Dalantercept is a soluble fusion protein of the extracellular domain of ALK-1 and human immunoglobulinG1 Fc that binds BMP9 and 10 and functions as a ligand trap.[13,14] Dalantercept inhibited angiogenesis in several preclinical model systems and was shown to enhance the efficacy of VEGFR TKI in RCC xenograft models.[15] Dalantercept was found to be tolerable in a phase 1study of solid tumors, with toxicities including fatigue, peripheral edema (dose limiting), anemia, nausea, and, at higher doses, cutaneous telangiectasias, which confirms the biologic relevance of the target (NCT00996957). A few objective responses and prolonged periods of stable disease were noted, supporting its clinical activity. Based on the preclinical data and single-agent early clinical data, dalantercept is currently being studied in combination with axitinib in patients with VEGFR TKI–resistant advanced RCC (NCT01642082).

Sphingosine-1-Phosphate

Sphingosine-1-phosphate (S1P) is a sphingolipid, pro-angiogenic signaling molecule that is generated by the activity of sphingosine-kinase-1 (SPHK1). S1P plays a role in the development of vascular networks and also inhibits apoptosis, potentiates motility and invasion of human tumor cell lines, and induces the secretion of cytokines such as IL-6 and IL-8, which are known to support tumor progression.[16] Overexpression of SPHK1 occurs in a variety of human cancers including RCC, and its expression is inversely associated with survival.[17] Upregulation of the oncogene, *sphk1*, and the resultant increase in S1P production and signaling in the tumor have been hypothesized to underlie resistance to multiple therapies including VEGF-directed anti-angiogenic treatment.

In a mouse human RCC xenograft model treated with sunitinib, SPHK1 was among the most highly upregulated genes that accompanied acquired resistance to VEGFR TKI therapy.[18] Plasma S1P was found to be at least 4-fold higher in patients with metastatic human RCC than in healthy controls, and S1P has been shown to increase with resistance to VEGFR TKI therapy in the majority of patients with advanced RCC. In RCC cell lines, S1P treatment led to IL-6 and IL-8 release, which was blocked by S1P antibody treatment. The anti-S1P antibody, sphingomab, also slowed RCC xenograft growth in treatment-naïve as well as sunitinib-resistant mice and was associated with a reduction in tumor blood flow, as measured by arterial spin-labeled magnetic resonance imaging.[18]

Drugs targeting the S1P axis include fingolimod, which is approved for multiple sclerosis, and a number of other compounds currently undergoing investigation in cancer (pancreatic, hematologic) and various neurodegenerative and immunologic conditions. Sonepcizumab (LT1009), a humanized anti-S1P antibody, is undergoing clinical investigation in patients with solid tumors (NCT00661414) and RCC (NCT01762033). The phase 1 study in advanced solid tumors yielded no dose-limiting toxicities and no drug-related serious adverse events, but infusion reactions occurred in three of nine patients at 24 mg/kg.[19] A few patients experienced long-term stable disease. The RCC study is an ongoing, phase 2, single-arm study in patients whose disease has progressed after at least three prior systemic therapies including VEGF pathway and mTOR inhibitors.

Human Double Minute 2: mdm2 Inhibitors

The oncoprotein human double minute 2 (HDM2; analogue of murine mdm2) is an E3 ubiquitin ligase involved in the negative regulation of p53 protein through ubiquitination, leading to proteasomal degradation. It also has non-p53–dependent actions that involve RNA and DNA synthesis, cell-cycle control, and cell membrane receptor regulation.[20] Downregulation of HDM2 leads to lower levels of hypoxia-inducible factor (HIF)-1 and HIF-2α in a p53- and VHL-independent manner.[21] Tumor cell p53 status is known to influence the tumor's sensitivity to angiogenesis inhibition and hypoxia-induced apoptosis.[22] p53 mutations are rare in RCC. In a mouse RCC xenograft model, sunitinib increased p53 levels, which then reverted to baseline simultaneously with the development of sunitinib resistance.[23] This resistance was associated with upregulation of HDM2 and perhaps, as a result, loss of expression of p53 downstream proteins, upregulation of HIF-2α, and tumor infiltration by CD11b+/Gr-1+ myeloid derived suppressor cells (MDSCs). In this model, the concurrent administration of MI-319, a HDM2/HDMX antagonist, was able to sustain the expression of p53 and significantly delay the onset of angiogenic escape pathways. Concomitant with delay in resistance, the HDM2 antagonist also prevented the enhanced expression of HIF-2α as well as the MDSC infiltration. Several HDM2 antagonists are currently undergoing clinical development.

Interleukin-8

In a human RCC xenograft model, resistance to sunitinib coincided with higher microvessel density, denoting escape from anti-angiogenic activity, and increased IL-8 secretion.[24] Sunitinib-resistant mice that were co-administered IL-8–neutralizing antibody had reduced tumor growth compared with mice that were continued on sunitinib alone or receiving only IL-8 antibody, consistent with a resensitizing effect of IL-8 antibody on VEGFR TKI resistance. In archival human clear-cell RCC (ccRCC) tissue, IL-8 expression was higher in patients who demonstrated intrinsic resistance to sunitinib than in responders, suggesting that preexisting IL-8 expression could contribute to early resistance to VEGFR TKI.[24] In a large phase 3 trial of pazopanib in patients with advanced RCC, higher levels of IL-8 were associated with shorter PFS.[25] Unfortunately, clinically applicable therapeutic strategies for targeting IL-8 currently do not exist.

Identifying Novel Targets That Lead to Early Resistance or Refractory Tumors

Hypoxia-Inducible Factor-2 alpha

In recent years, HIF-2α has emerged as the more relevant HIF in the development and progression of RCC. Initial studies showed that inhibition of HIF-2α is sufficient for suppression of tumor growth in VHL-defective RCC cell lines.[26] Additional experiments have suggested that HIF-1α may function as a tumor suppressor in VHL-null RCC.[27] In particular, tumor-promoting genes that encode cyclin D1, TGF-α, and VEGF have been shown to be driven specifically by HIF-2α, with differential effects of HIF-1α (growth retarding) and HIF-2α (growth promoting) observed in RCC tumor xenografts.[28] Indeed, up to 40% of RCCs have deletions in the HIF1α-containing portion of chromosome 14q,[29] and RCC expressing only HIF-2 appears to exhibit a more aggressive clinical behavior.[30]

While laboratory effects of chemical and biological inhibitors of HIF-2α on tumor cells are being investigated,[31] clinical grade HIF-2α–specific inhibitors have yet to be developed. In the meantime, evaluation of approaches that nonspecifically block HIF-2α, such as the HDM2 antagonists mentioned previously or the target of rapamycin complex (TORC2) inhibitors (see below), merit exploration.

Mammalian Target of Rapamycin Complex 1 and 2 and Phosphatidyl Inositol 3 Kinase

The currently approved inhibitors of mTOR, everolimus and temsirolimus, primarily inhibit TORC1, the complex that includes mTOR and raptor (regulatory associated protein of TOR), and have less activity against TORC2, the complex that includes mTOR and rictor (the rapamycin-insensitive companion of TOR). The translation of HIF-2α, the dominant oncogene in RCC, is more dependent on the activity of TORC2 and largely independent of the TORC1 activity.[32] A potential mechanism for acquired resistance to mTORC1 inhibitors is loss of negative feedback loops that are normally operative when mTORC1 is active, such as suppression of mTORC2 and its activation of AKT, resulting in the upregulation of HIF.[33] A TORC-dependent negative feedback loop also involves activation of upstream receptor tyrosine kinases such as insulin-like growth factor I receptors (IGF-IR)/phosphatidyl inositol 3 kinase(PI3K)/AKT signaling, which may also lead to therapeutic resistance. These findings highlight the potential for dual TORC1 and 2 inhibition in RCC as a strategy to limit acquired resistance to TORC1 inhibitors.

A new generation of dual mTOR inhibitors that bind directly to the ATP-binding domain of mTOR, blocking both TORC1 and TORC2 activity including HIF-2α expression, is under development.[34] Several novel dual mTORC1/2 inhibitors have been studied in cell-line– and tumor xenograft–based preclinical models. In a phase 1 trial of a PI3K inhibitor, BKM120, 28 of 66 patients with non-RCC solid tumors exhibited antitumor benefit, including 2 partial responses and 18 metabolic responses.[35] This agent is now being tested in combination with bevacizumab in patients with advanced RCC (NCT01283048). BEZ235 showed enhanced efficacy relative to rapamycin in RCC xenograft models.[36] Efforts to develop this agent clinically in RCC and other cancers, however, have been stymied by significant side effects. Another approach involves GDC-0980, a dual PI3K/mTORC1/2 inhibitor that appears to be better tolerated than BEZ235. A randomized phase 2 trial of GDC-980 versus everolimus has been conducted (NCT01442090) with results pending.

Neurofibromin 2, Merlin, and Hippo Pathway

Neurofibromin 2 (*NF2*) loss is known to predispose to neurofibromatosis II and benign neural tumors. In a whole-genome sequencing study of a large cohort of primary RCC tumors and cell lines, it was found that a significant fraction (33%) of VHL wild-type (WT) ccRCCs contained inactivating mutations of the tumor suppressor gene *NF2*.[37] Further, knockout of *NF2* in mouse kidney epithelium has been shown to lead to the development of invasive RCC, thus confirming a causal role of *NF2* inactivation in RCC.[38]

Merlin, the protein product of *NF2*, has been identified through genetic studies as an upstream regulator of the Hippo signaling pathway.[39,40] The Hippo pathway appears to be a critical growth regulatory pathway that is deregulated in many types of human cancers.[41] It is composed of a core kinase cascade that phosphorylates and inhibits the oncoprotein Yap.

Recent data suggest that the Hippo pathway may also be inactivated in a significant percentage of VHL null RCC, leading to Yap nuclear translocation and activation. For example, *WW45/SAV1*, which is located on 14q22.1, has been found to be downregulated in 72% of high-grade ccRCC.[42] Significantly, it was shown in the same study that the levels of WW45 inversely correlated with the amount of nuclear Yap, and as much as 58% of high-grade ccRCC exhibited primarily nuclear Yap staining. Although efforts to target the downstream effects of *NF2* and Hippo pathway loss and Yap activation in human cancer are nascent and its relevance to RCC remains to be fully elucidated, exploration of this signaling network may provide crucial insights into RCC biology and identify therapeutic targets for at least a subset of patients with either VHL-WT or VHL-null RCC.

Future Approaches to Optimize Initial Therapy of Renal Cell Carcinoma

At a population level, reduction in the burden of RCC will rely on prevention, early detection, and effective adjuvant therapy after surgical resection, as well as control and/or cure of advanced disease with interventions that have an improved therapeutic index. It is anticipated that improved understanding of the biology of RCC will continue to contribute to progress in the management of patients with advanced disease. As described above, such biologic insights are coming from a better understanding of the mechanisms of resistance to VEGF inhibitors, a better understanding of the interplay between the tumor and the immune microenvironment, and analyses of novel mechanisms that drive RCC and are identified through analyses such as TCGA. In particular, TCGA carries significant potential to identify driver mutations and pathways that have the potential for therapeutic targeting, either in individual cases or as part of a new molecularly based classification of RCC.[43] Examples that are already being explored include the chromatin modifiers, PI3K-mTOR pathway activators, and pathways mediated by *NF2* loss. The application of genetic, immunologic, or other biomarkers that result from such research has the potential to select patients with specific tumor types for therapy targeted to specific vulnerabilities, resistance mechanisms, or sensitivities within their tumor and/or microenvironment. Such advances should enable an era of rational and more effective therapy for patients with advanced RCC.

References

1. Yamakawa M, Liu LX, Belanger AJ, et al. Expression of angiopoietins in renal epithelial and clear cell carcinoma cells: regulation by hypoxia and participation in angiogenesis. *Am J Physiol Renal Physiol.* 2004;287(4):F649–F657.

2. Huang J, Bae JO, Tsai JP, et al. Angiopoietin-1/Tie-2 activation contributes to vascular survival and tumor growth during VEGF blockade. *Int J Oncol.* 2009;34(1):79–87.

3. Kienast Y, Christian K, Scheuer W, et al. Ang-2-VEGF-A CrossMab, a novel bispecific human IgG1 antibody blocking VEGF-A and Ang-2 functions simultaneously, mediates potent anti-tumor, anti-angiogenic, and anti-metastatic efficacy. *Clin Cancer Res.* 2013;19:6730–6740.

4. Rini B, Szczylik C, Tannir NM, et al. AMG 386 in combination with sorafenib in patients with metastatic clear cell carcinoma of the kidney: a randomized, double-blind, placebo-controlled, phase 2 study. *Cancer.* 2012;118:6152–6161.

5. Atkins MB, Ravaud A, Gravis G, et al. Safety and efficacy of AMG 386 in combination with sunitinib in patients with metastatic renal cell carcinoma (mRCC) in an open-label multicenter phase II study. *J Clin Oncol*.2012;30(suppl; abstr 4606).

6. Pennacchietti S, Michieli P, Galluzzo M, Mazzone M, Giordano S, Comoglio PM. Hypoxia promotes invasive growth by transcriptional activation of the met protooncogene. *Cancer Cell*.2003;3(4):347–361.

7. Koochekpour S, Jeffers M, Wang PH, et al. The von Hippel-Lindau tumor suppressor gene inhibits hepatocyte growth factor/ scatter factor-induced invasion and branching morphogenesis in renal carcinoma cells. *Mol Cel Biol*.1999;19(9):5902–5912.

8. Gibney G, Conrad P, Aziz SA, et al. C-met as a therapeutic target using ARQ 197 in renal cell carcinoma. *J Clin Oncol*. 2011; 2009: abstr 360.

9. Shojaei F, Lee JH, Simmons BH, et al. HGF/c-Met acts as an alternate angiogenic pathway in sunitinib resistant tumors. *Cancer Res*. 2010;70:10090–10100.

10. Michael Yakes F, Chen J, Tan J, et al. Cabozantinib (XL184), a novel MET and VEGFR2 inhibitor, simultaneously suppresses metastasis, angiogenesis, and tumor growth. *Mol Cancer Ther*. 2011;10;2298–2308.

11. Choueiri TK, Pal SK, McDermott DF, et al. Efficacy of cabozantinib in patients with metastatic refractory renal carcinoma (RCC). *J Clin Oncol*. 2012;30 (abstr 4504).

12. Eder JP, Vande Woude GF, Boerner SA et al. Novel therapeutic inhibitors of the c-Met signaling pathway in cancer. *Clin Cancer Res*. 2009;15:2207–2214.

13. Mitchell D, Pobre E, Mulivor A, et al. ALK-1-Fc inhibits multiple mediators of angiogenesis and suppresses tumor growth. *Mol Cancer Ther*. 2010;9:379–388.

14. Van Meeteren LA, Thorikay M, Bergqvist S, et al. Anti-human activin receptor-like kinase 1 (ALK-1) antibody attenuates bone morphogenetic protein 9 (BMP9)-induced ALK-1 signaling and interferes with endothelial cell sprouting. *J Biol Chem*. 2012;287:18551–18561.

15. WangX, SolbanN, BhasinMK, et al. ALK1-Fc inhibits tumor growth in a VEGF pathway resistance model of renal cell carcinoma. *Cancer Res*. 2012;72(8 suppl): AbstractLB-313.

16. Kunkel GT, Maceyka M, Milstien S, et al. Targeting the sphingosine-1-phosphate axis in cancer, inflammation and beyond. *Nat Rev Drug Discov*. 2013;12:688–702.

17. Facchinetti MM, Gandini NA, Fermento ME. The expression of sphingosine kinase-1 in head and neck carcinoma. *Cells Tissues Organs*. 2010;192:314–324.

18. Bhatt RS, Zhang L, Bullock A, et al. Sphingosine-1-phosphate (S1P) as a novel target in renal cancer (RCC) In: Proceedings of the 101st Annual Meeting of the American Association for Cancer Research; April 17–21, 2010; Washington, DC. AACR. Abstract LB-369/8.

19. Gordon MS, Just R, Rosen LS, et al. A phase I study of sonepcizumab (S), a humanized monoclonal antibody to sphingosine-1-phosphate (S1P), in patients with advanced solid tumors. *J Clin Oncol*.2010;28:15s(suppl; abstr 2560).

20. Zhang Z, Zhang R. p53-independent activities of MDM2and their relevance to cancer therapy. *Curr Cancer Drug Targets*. 2005;5:9–20.

21. Carroll VA, Ashcroft M. Regulation of angiogenic factors by HDM2 in renal cell carcinoma. *Cancer Res*. 2008;68:545–552.

22. Yu JL, Rak JW, Coomber BL, et al: Effect of p53 status on tumor response to antiangiogenic therapy. *Science*. 2002,295:1526–1528.

23. Panka DJ, Liu Q, Geissler AK, et al. Effects of HDM2 antagonism on sunitinib resistance, p53 activation, SDF-1 induction, and tumor infiltration by
CD11b+/Gr-1+ myeloid derived suppressor cells. *Mol Cancer.* 2013;12:1–12.

24. Huang D, Ding Y, Zhou M, et al. Interleukin-8 mediates resistance to antiangiogenic agent sunitinib in renal cell carcinoma. *Cancer Res.* 2010;70:1063–1071.

25. Liu Y, Tran HT, Lin Y, et al: Plasma cytokine and angiogenic factors (CAFs)
predictive of clinical benefit and prognosis in patients (Pts) with advanced or
metastatic renal cell cancer (mRCC) treated in phase III trials of pazopanib
(PAZO). *J Clin Oncol.*2011;29: (suppl 7; abstr 334).

26. Kondo K, Kim WY, Lechpammer M, Kaelin WG Jr. Inhibition of HIF2α
is sufficient to suppress pVHL-defective tumor growth. *PLoS Biol.*
2003;1(3):e83.

27. Shen C, Beroukhim R, Schumaker SE et al. Genetic and functional studies
implicate HIF1α as a 14q kidney cancer suppressor gene. *Cancer Discovery.*
2011;1:222–235.

28. Raval RR, Lau KW, Tran MG, et al. Contrasting properties of hypoxia-inducible
factor 1 (HIF-1) and HIF-2 in von Hippel-Lindau-associated renal cell carcinoma. *Mol Cell Biol.* 2005;25:5675–5686.

29. Beroukhim R, Brunet JP, Di Napoli A, et al. Patterns of gene expression and
copy-number alterations in vonHippel–Lindau disease-associated and sporadic clear cell carcinoma of the kidney. *Cancer Res.* 2009;69:4674–4681.

30. Gordan JD, Lal P, Dondeti VR, et al. HIF-α effects on c-Myc distinguish two
subtypes of sporadic VHL-deficient clear cell renal carcinoma. *Cancer Cell.*
2008;14:435–446.

31. Zimmer M, Ebert BL, Neil C, et al. Small-molecule inhibitors of HIF-2a translation link its 5'UTR iron-responsive element to oxygen sensing. *Mol Cell.*
2008;32:838–848.

32. Toschi A, Lee E, Gadir N, et al. Differential dependence of hypoxia-inducible
factors 1 alpha and 2 alpha on TORC1 and TORC2. *J Biol Chem.*
2008;283:34495–34499.

33. O'Reilly KE, Rojo F, She QB, et al. mTOR inhibition induces upstream receptor
tyrosine kinase signaling and activates akt. *Cancer Res.*2006;66:1500–1508.

34. Figlin RA, Kaufmann I, Brechbiel J. Targeting PI3K and mTORC2 in metastatic
renal cell carcinoma: new strategies for overcoming resistance to VEGFR and
mTORC1 inhibitors. *Int J Cancer.* 2013;133:788–796.

35. Burris H, Rodon J, S. Sharma S, et al. First-in-human phase I study of the oral
PI3K inhibitor BEZ235 in patients (pts) with advanced solid tumors. *J Clin
Oncol.* 2010;28 (suppl): 3005

36. Cho DC, Cohen MB, Panka DJ, et al. The efficacy of the novel dual PI3-kinase/
mTOR inhibitor NVP-BEZ235 compared with rapamycin in renal cell carcinoma. *Clin Cancer Res.* 2010;16:3628–3638.

37. Dalgliesh GL, Furge K, Greenman C, et al. Systematic sequencing of
renal carcinoma reveals inactivation of histone modifying genes. *Nature.*
2010;463:360–363.

38. Morris ZS, McClatchey AI. Aberrant epithelial morphology and persistent epi-
dermal growth factor receptor signaling in a mouse model of renal carcinoma.
Proc Natl Acad Sci U S A. 2009;106:9767–9772.

39. Zhang N, et al. The Merlin/NF2 tumor suppressor functions through the YAP
oncoprotein to regulate tissue homeostasis in mammals. *Developmental Cell.*
2010;19:27–38.

40. Hamaratoglu F, et al., The tumour-suppressor genes NF2/Merlin and Expanded act through Hippo signalling to regulate cell proliferation and apoptosis. *Nature Cell Biol*. 2006;8:27–36.

41. Harvey KF, Zhang X, Thomas DM. The Hippo pathway and human cancer. *Nat Rev Cancer*. 2013;13:246–257.

42. Matsuura K, Nakada C, Mashio M, et al. Downregulation of SAV1 plays a role in pathogenesis of high-grade clear cell renal cell carcinoma. *BMC Cancer*. 2011;11: 523.

43. Choueiri TK, Pomerantz MM, Signoretti S. Renal-cell carcinoma: a step closer to a new classification. *Lancet Oncol*. 2013;14:105–107.

Index

Page numbers followed by t indicate a table on the designated page

A

acquired cystic disease-associated RCC, 10t, 14

active surveillance methods, 47–48, 49t–50t

acupuncture, 166t, 168, 169–170,

Adjuvant Sorafenib or Sunitinib for Unfavorable Renal Carcinoma (ASSURE) study, 64, 65

adverse events (AEs), in mRCC
  interferon-α plus bevacizumab, 133, 134t–136t
  manifestations and management
    hyperlipidemia, 144
    hypertension, 144
    mucositis, 137
    pneumonitis, 144
    rash, 137
    renal issues, 144–145
  mTOR inhibitors, 134t–136t, 137
  tyrosine kinase inhibitors, 133, 134t–136t, 137

AGS-003 dendritic cell-based vaccine, 85

Akt predictive biomarker, of mTOR pathway, 126

alcohol consumption, 4

ALK-1 (activin-like kinase-1) inhibitors, 176t, 177t, 179. See also crizotinib; dalantercept; PF-03446962

allogenic stem cell transplantation, 85

American Cancer Society (ACS) Prevention Study, 170

amitriptyline, 158t

ancillary tests, for RCC classification, 16

angiomyolipomas (AMLs), 21, 32

angiopoietins, 175, 176t, 178

Armstrong, A. J., 126

AURKA (aurora kinase A) inhibitors, 21

axitinib (tyrosine kinase inhibitor), 90t
  adjuvant therapy, 64, 66t
  adverse effects in mRCC, 134t, 136t
  for metastatic clear-cell RCC, 90t, 95t, 100t, 101, 104t, 106
  for VEGFR TKI-resistant advanced RCC, 179

B

bacille Calmette-Guérin vaccine, 62, 64

BAP1 mutation nonvalidated biomarker, 123t, 126

bevacizumab, 84
  adverse events from, 133, 134t, 136t, 137, 144–145
    management of, 141t, 142t, 143t
  with IFN-alpha, 82, 90t, 133
    adverse events, 133
  for metastatic clear-cell RCC, 89, 90t, 93t, 94t, 96t, 97t, 100t, 104t, 105t
  for sarcomatoid RCC, 112

biology of RCC, 19–23, 47
  ccRCC, secondary mutations of chromatin remodeling genes, 21–22
  clear cell RCC tumors, 118
  improvements in understanding, 71, 85, 183
  mammalian target of rapamycin pathway, 21, 95
  RCC as a metabolic disease, 22
  relevant drug discoveries, 117
  research successes, 128
  von Hippel-Landau pathway, 19–21, 20f

biomarkers. See predictive biomarkers; prognostic biomarkers

Birt-Hogg-Dubé (BHD) syndrome, 28, 30–31, 33, 111

Brahmer, J. R., 83

breast cancer 1 (BRCA1)-associated protein-1 (BAP1) mutation, 32–33

C

c-MET inhibitors, 178, 179

c-MET/HGF (hepatocyte growth factor) pathway, 178

cabozantinib (XL184), 176t, 178–179

CAM. See complementary and alternative medicine

cancer-related fatigue (CRF), 155, 159

carcinoma associated with neuroblastoma, 13

carcinoma of the collecting ducts of Bellini, 10

CARMENA trial, 76

Centers for Epidemiologic Studies-Depression scale, 161

checkpoint blockade therapies, 7–8

Choueiri, T. K., 75

chromophobe renal cell carcinoma (ChRCC)
  description, 12
  morphological features, immunohistochemical profile, 11t
  systemic therapy, 110–112
  tumor necrosis in, 15
  WHO classification, 10t

chromosomes 9p and 14q deletions, nonvalidated biomarkers, 123t, 125–126

chronic obstructive pulmonary disease (COPD), 3